Exercises in Radiological Diagnosis

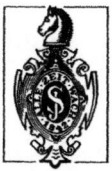

Michel Runge

Bones and Joints

170 Radiological Exercises for Students and Practitioners

With 407 Illustrations

Springer-Verlag
Berlin Heidelberg New York
London Paris Tokyo

Dr. MICHEL RUNGE

Centre Hospitalier et Universitaire de Besançon
Unité de Radiologie Ostéo-Articulaire
Hôpital Jean Minjoz
Boulevard Fleming

F-25030 Besançon

Translated from the French by

MARIE-THÉRÈSE WACKENHEIM

ISBN 978-3-540-16544-6   ISBN 978-3-642-85818-5 (eBook)
DOI 10.1007/978-3-642-85818-5

Library of Congress Cataloging-in-Publication Data. Runge, Michel, 1949- Bones and joints. (Exercises in radiological diagnosis) Translation of: Os et articulations. Bibliography: p. Includes index. 1. Bones–Radiography–Problems, exercises, etc. 2. Joints–Radiography–Problems, exercises, etc. 3. Bones–Diseases–Diagnosis–Atlases. 4. Joints–Diseases–Diagnosis–Atlases. I. Title. II. Series. [DNLM: 1. Bone and Bones–radiography–examination questions. 2. Joints–radiography–examination question. WE 18 R9420] RC930.5.R8613 1987 616.7'10757'076 86-31650
ISBN 978-3-540-16544-6

The use of registered names, trademarks, etc. in this publication does not imply, even in the absence of a specific statement, that such names are exempt from the relevant protective laws and regulations and therefore free for general use.

Product Liability: The publisher can give no guarantee for information about drug dosage and application there of contained in this book. In every individual case the respective user must check its accuracy by consulting other pharmaceutical literature.

2127/3130-543210

Forword

Conventional radiography of the bones and joints is holding its own brilliantly against the new imaging techniques. This is true although endoscopy has demoralized the adepts of barium sulfate, ultrasonography has eliminated radiologic investigations as solidly anchored as cholecystography, computer tomography (CT) has become prominent in the study of the retroperitoneal space and magnetic resonance imaging of the spinal cord already ridicules myelography. Standard radiography of the bones actually remains the most practical, quickest, cheapest, and often even the most precise procedure. Although CT now often replaces conventional tomography, CT scanning and magnetic resonance imaging are, in this field, still regarded as complimentary investigations. Interpretation of what are still sometimes called plain films is, in fact, often difficult. Anatomical variants and degenerative, traumatic, tumoral and infective lesions are intercrossed, superimposed, and form a tangle, compelling the radiologist to undertake the delicate task of disentangling them.

Michel Runge's book of exercises concerning the radiology of bones and joints really confronts a present-day problem. In the spirit of this remarkable series directed by Professor A. Wackenheim, Michel Runge has conceived and realized this book as a game aimed at simultaneously entertaining and enriching. There is no doubt that the reader/player will appreciate it.

J. F. BONNEVILLE

Contents

Introduction

Osteoarticular pathology is a very frequent motive for consultation. Very often, the diagnosis relies upon symptomatology, and the physician requires confirmatory radiological investigations. Whatever the clinical indication, the interpretation of radiological data must be very rigorous. On the basis of a complete description of the radiographic images, according to a systematic analysis plan, a certain number of diagnostic hypotheses may be proposed.

Selection of the most likely hypothesis requires the correlation of clinical, biological, and radiological data, and may sometimes necessitate additional investigations, such as tomograms, scintigrams, and computed tomography (CT).

Part One

Iconography

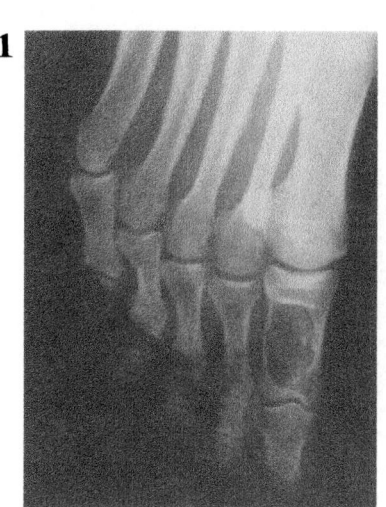

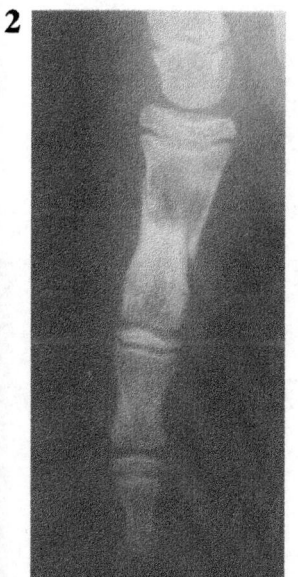

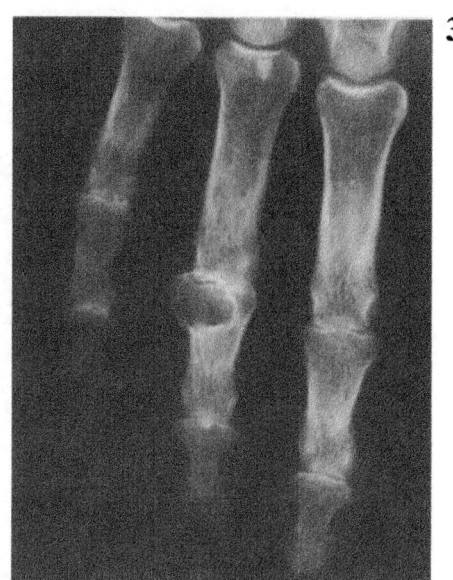

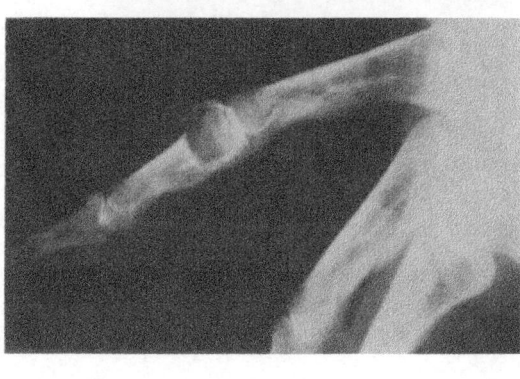

5
6

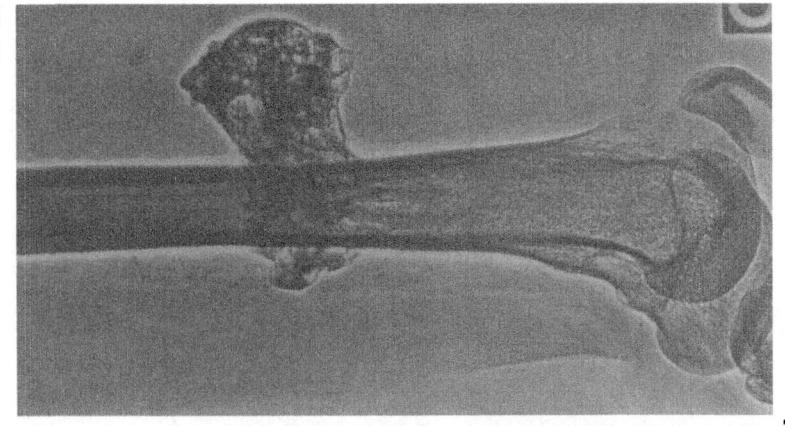

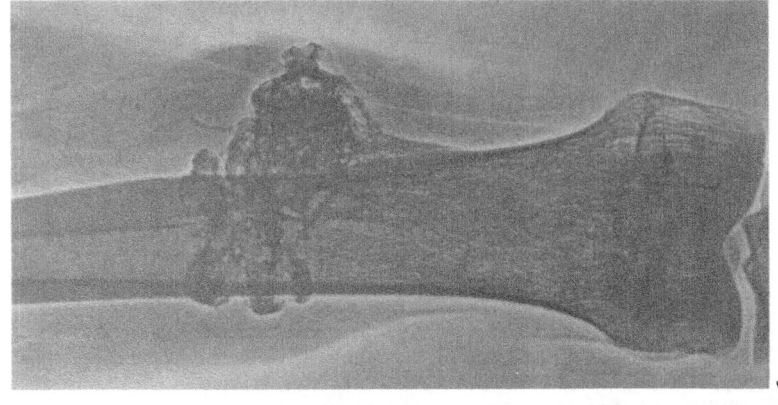

6a

5

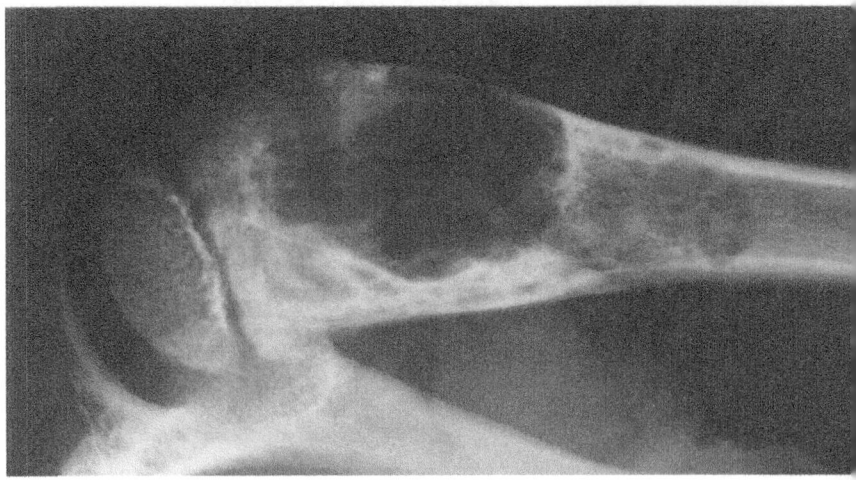

b

6

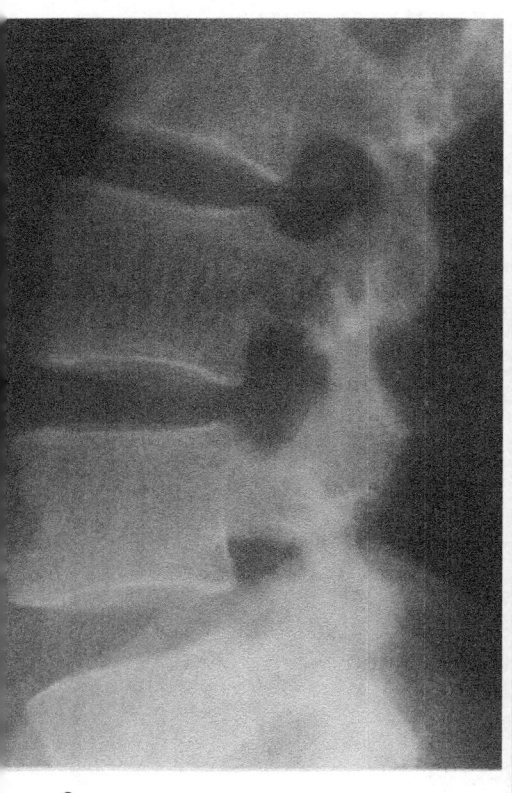

a

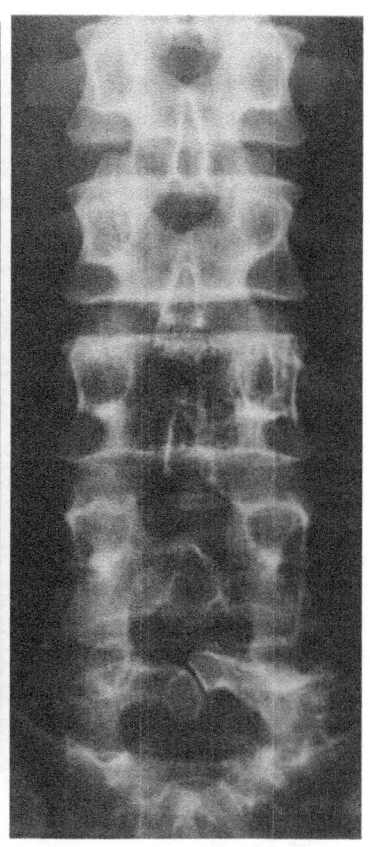

b

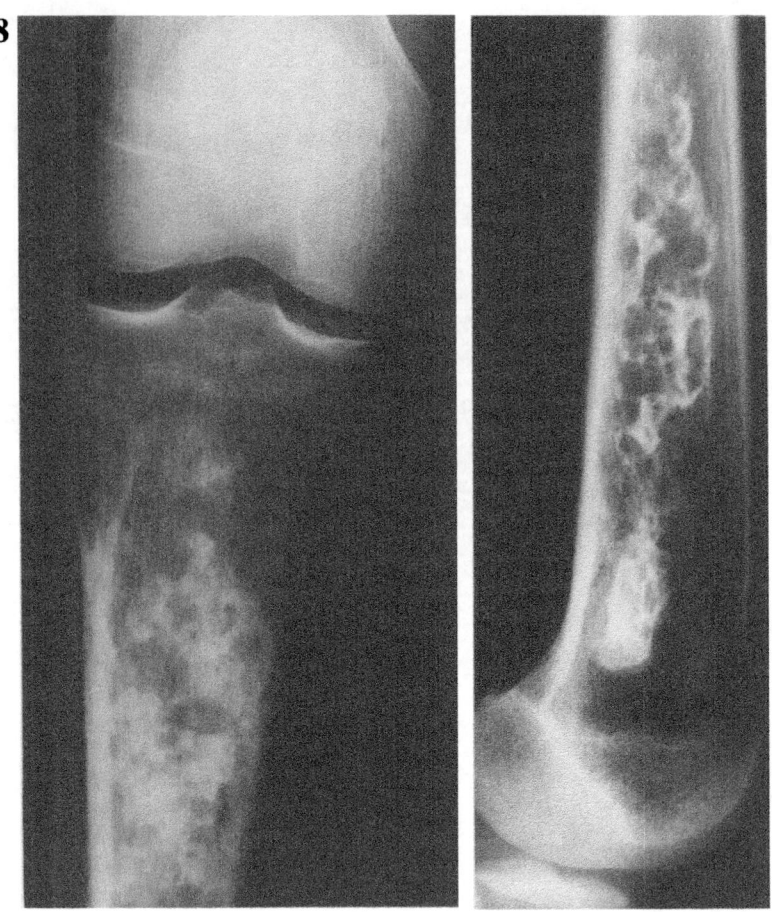

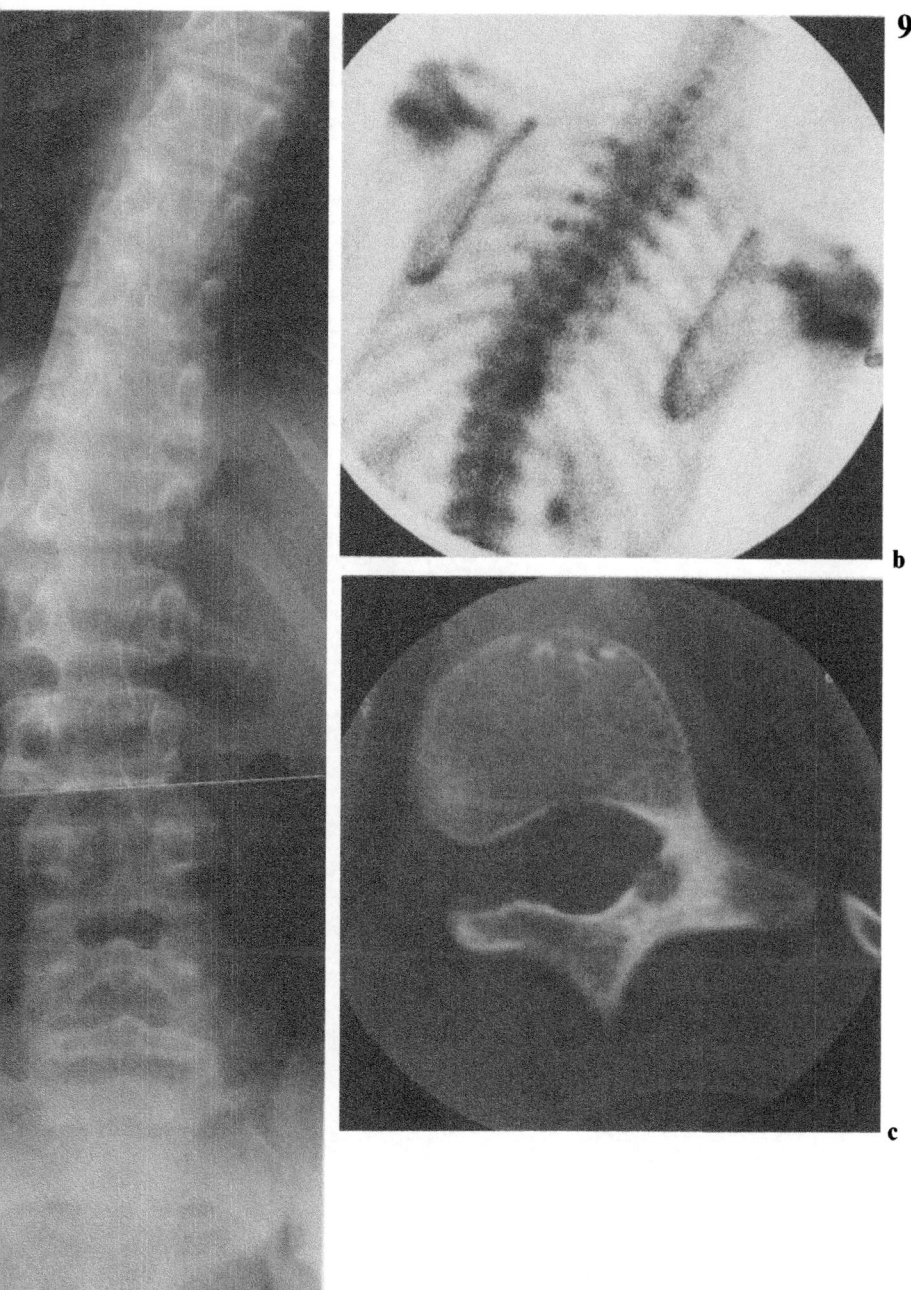

a

b

c

10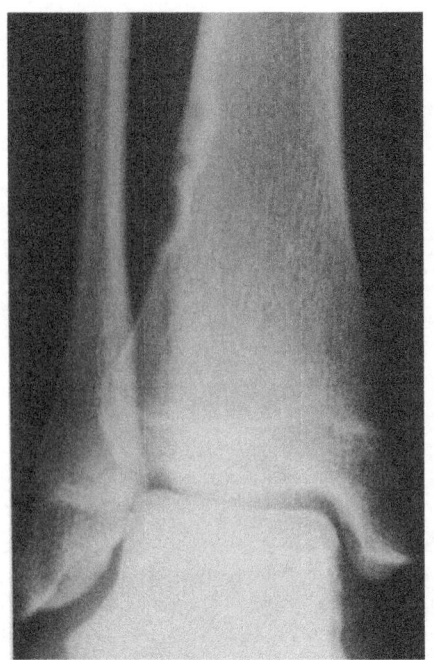

11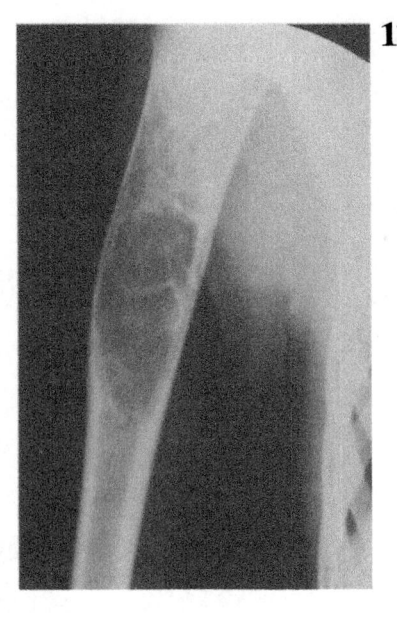

12

13

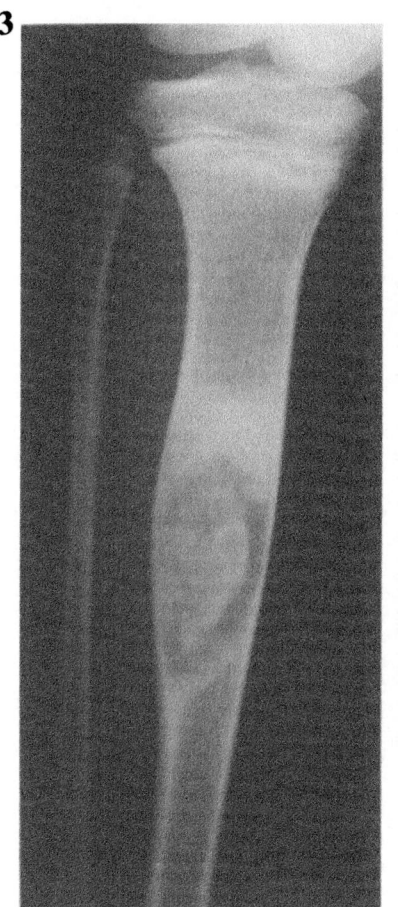

14

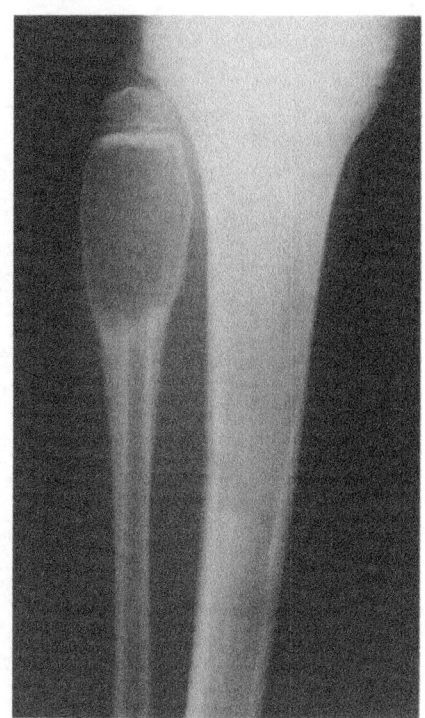

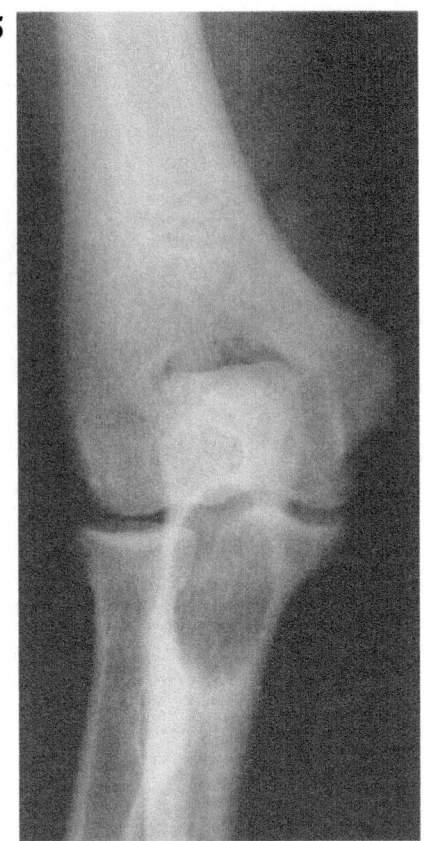

a

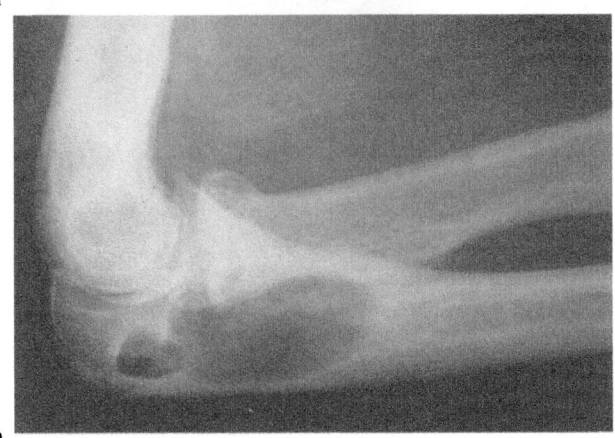

b

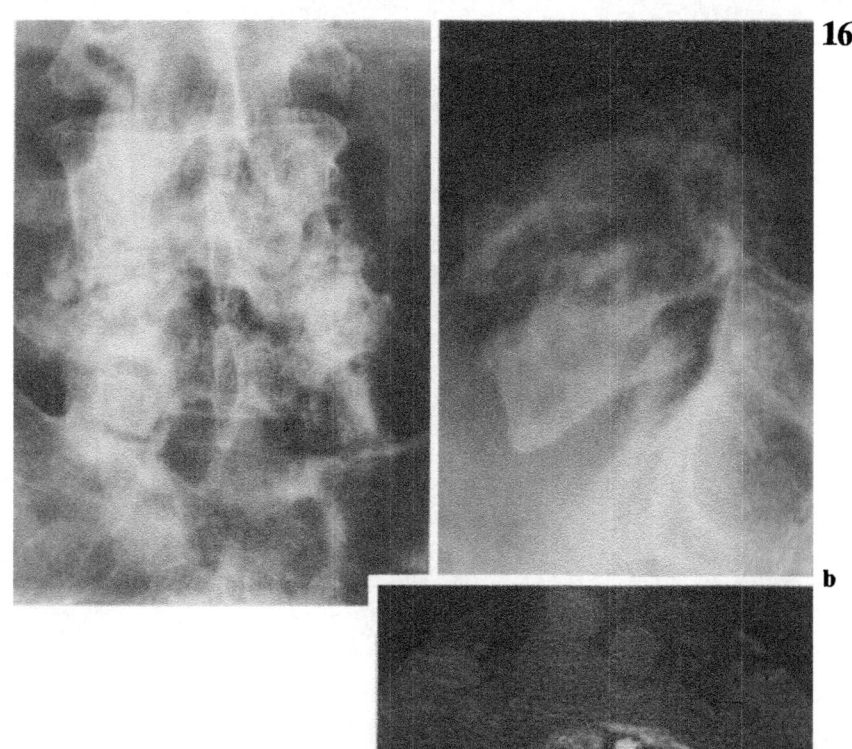

a

b

c

17

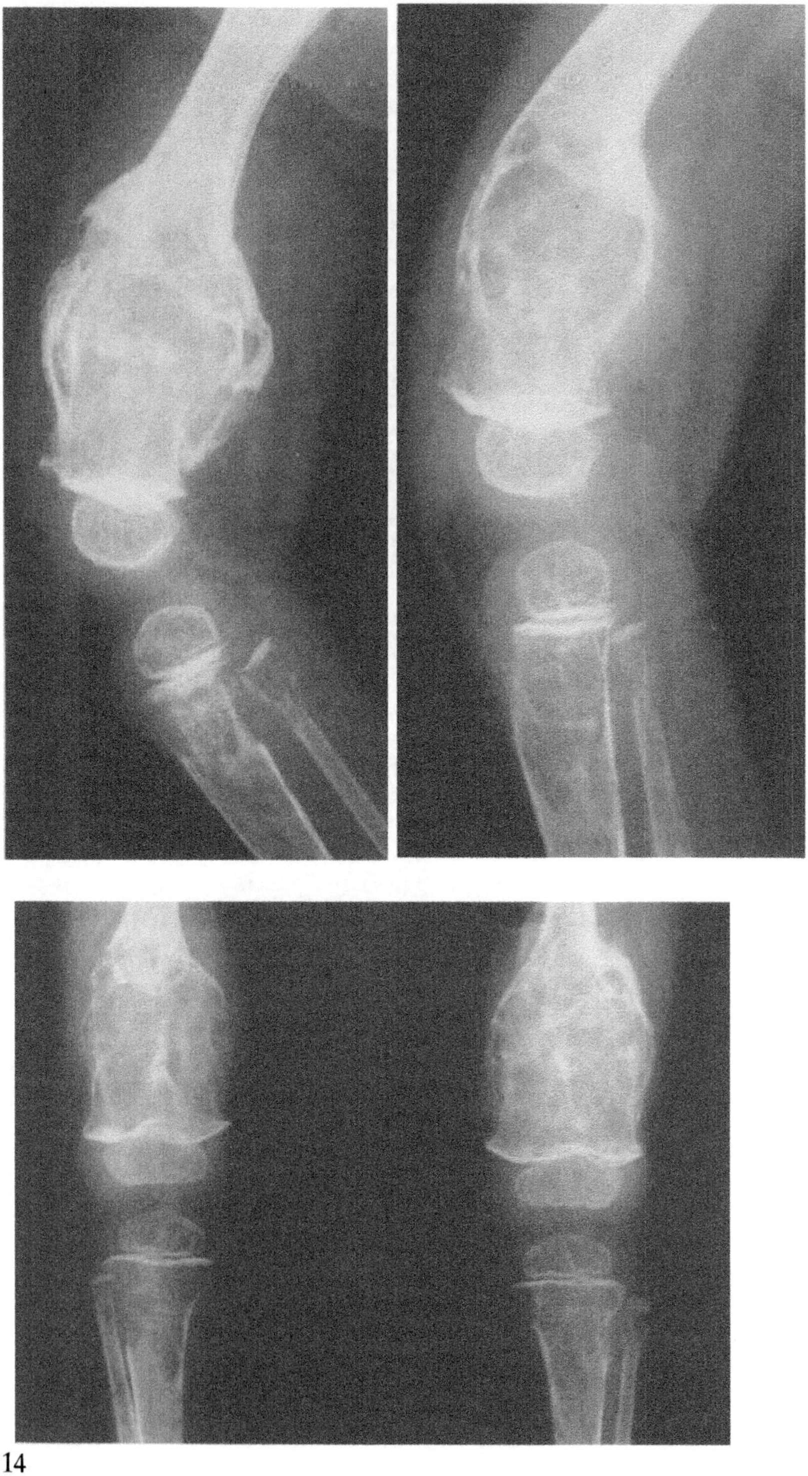

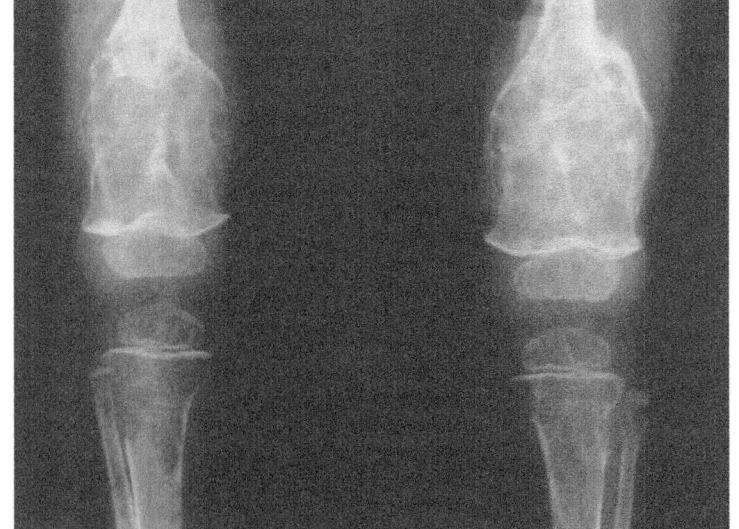

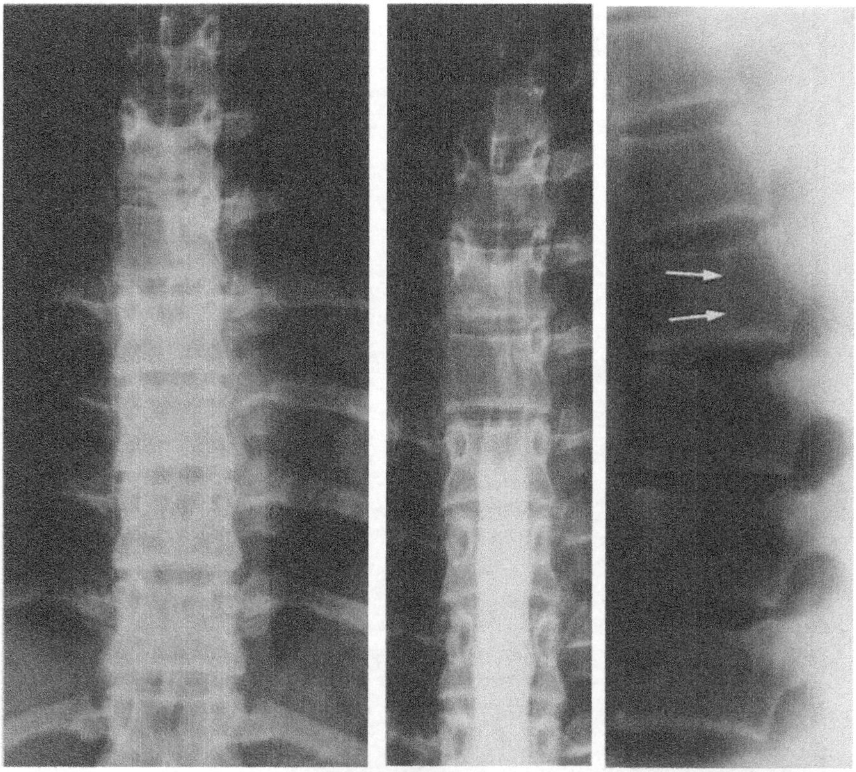

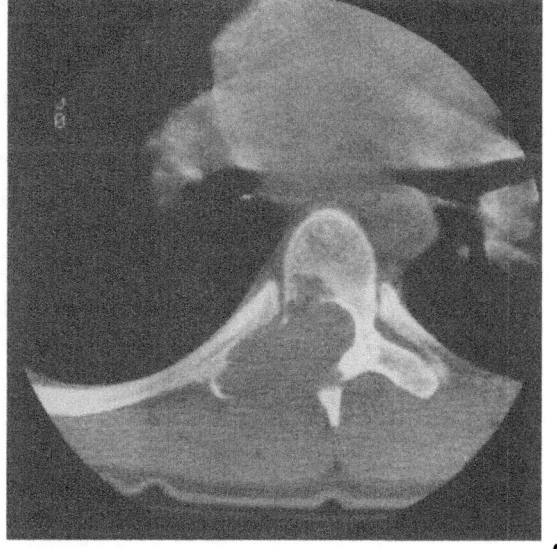

a

b,c

d

19

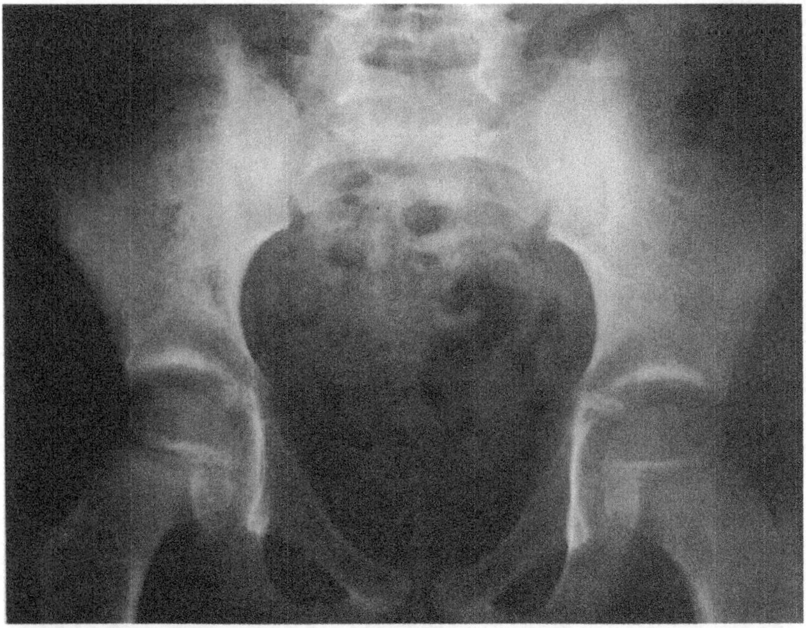

a

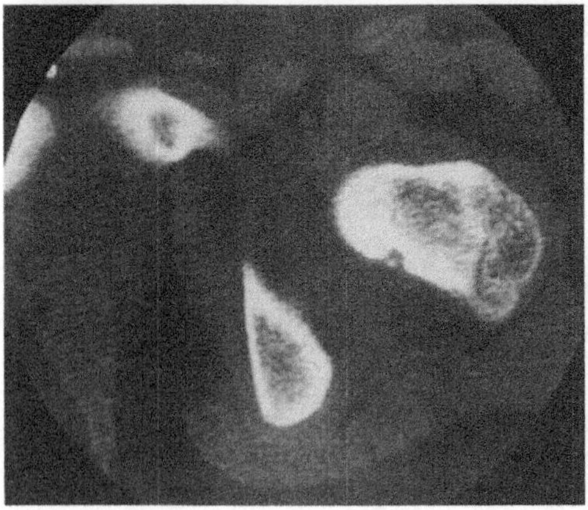

b

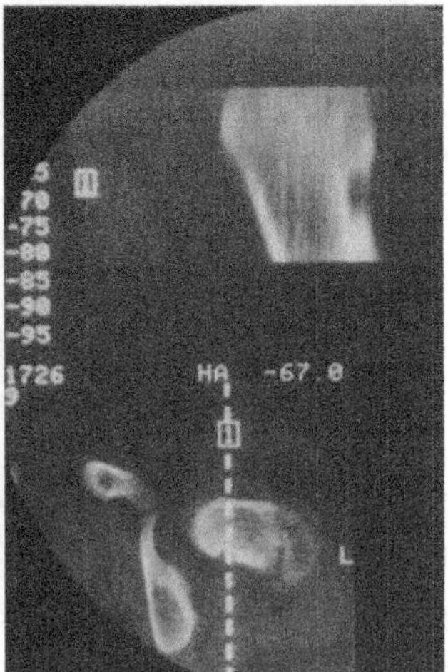

c

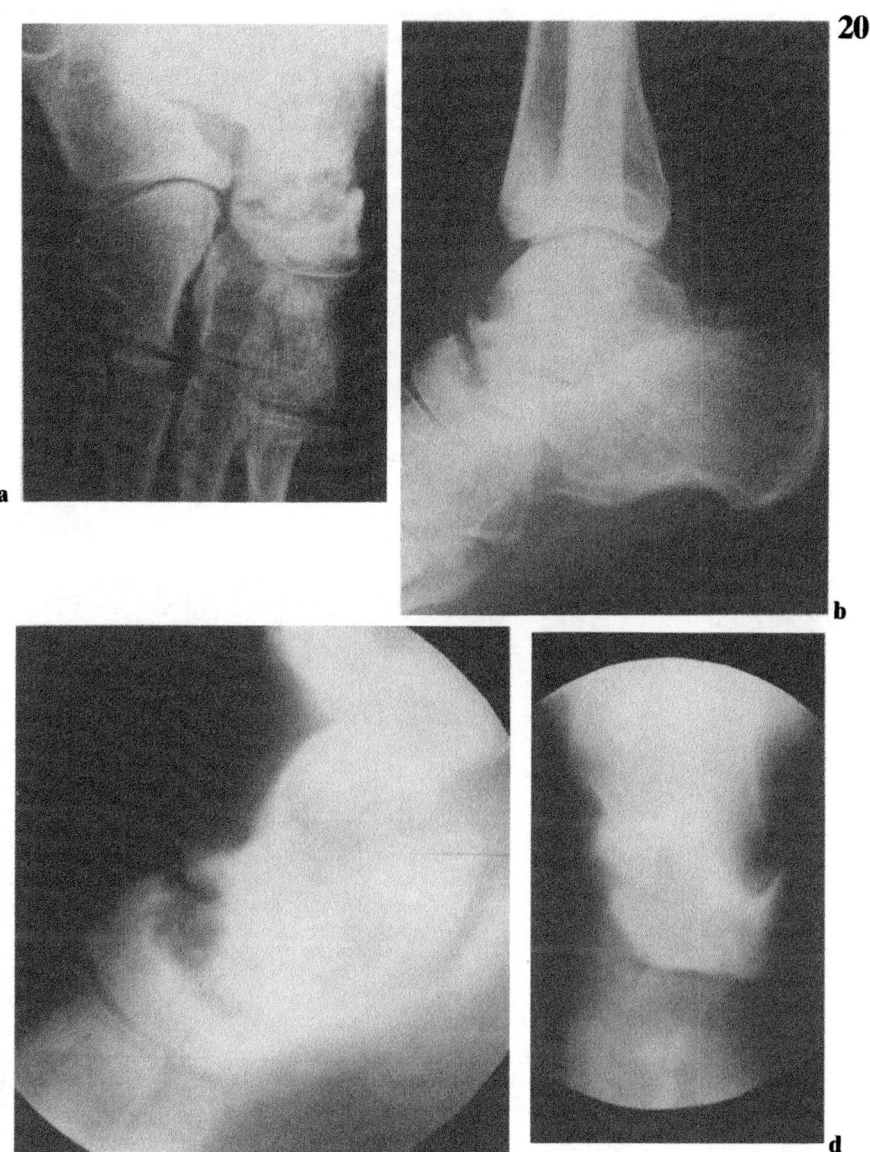

a

b

c

d

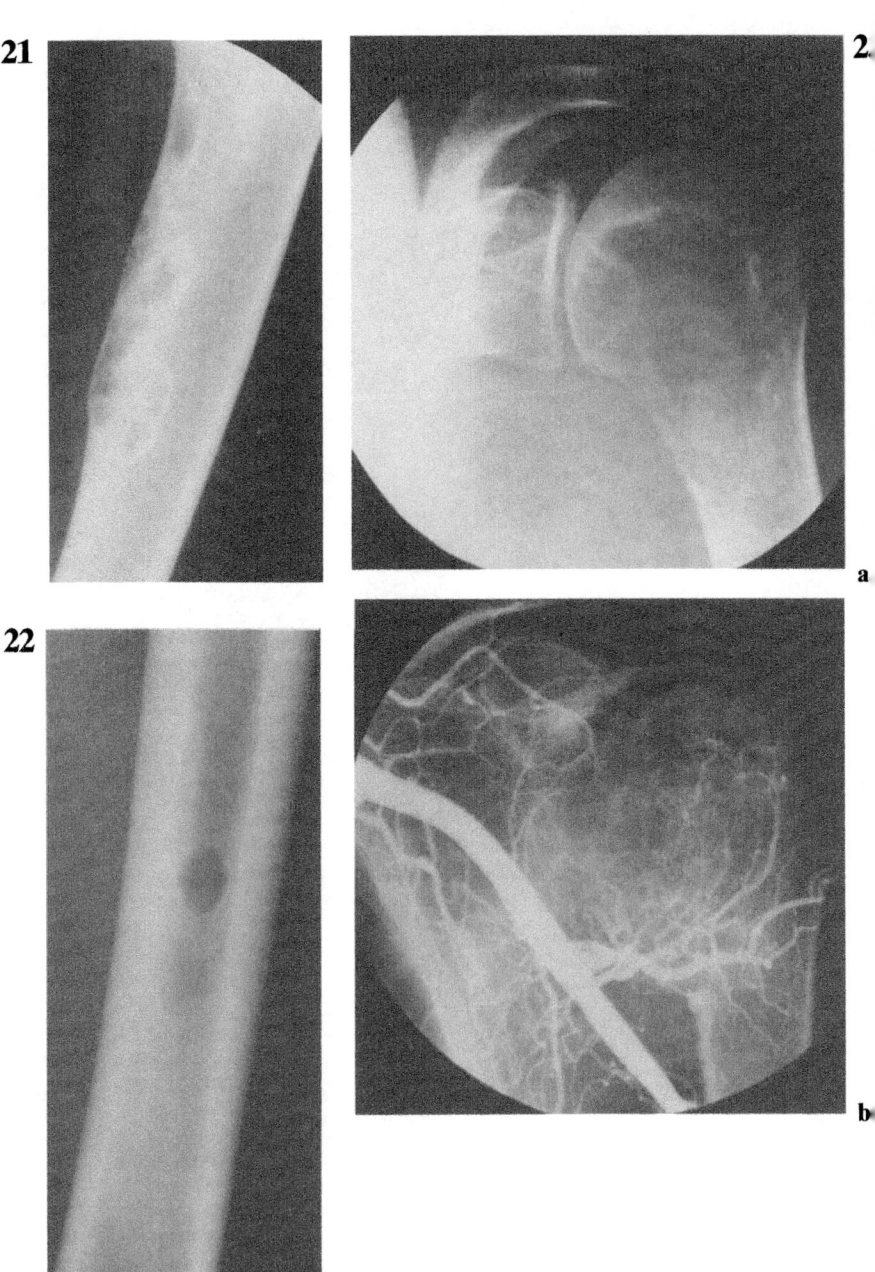

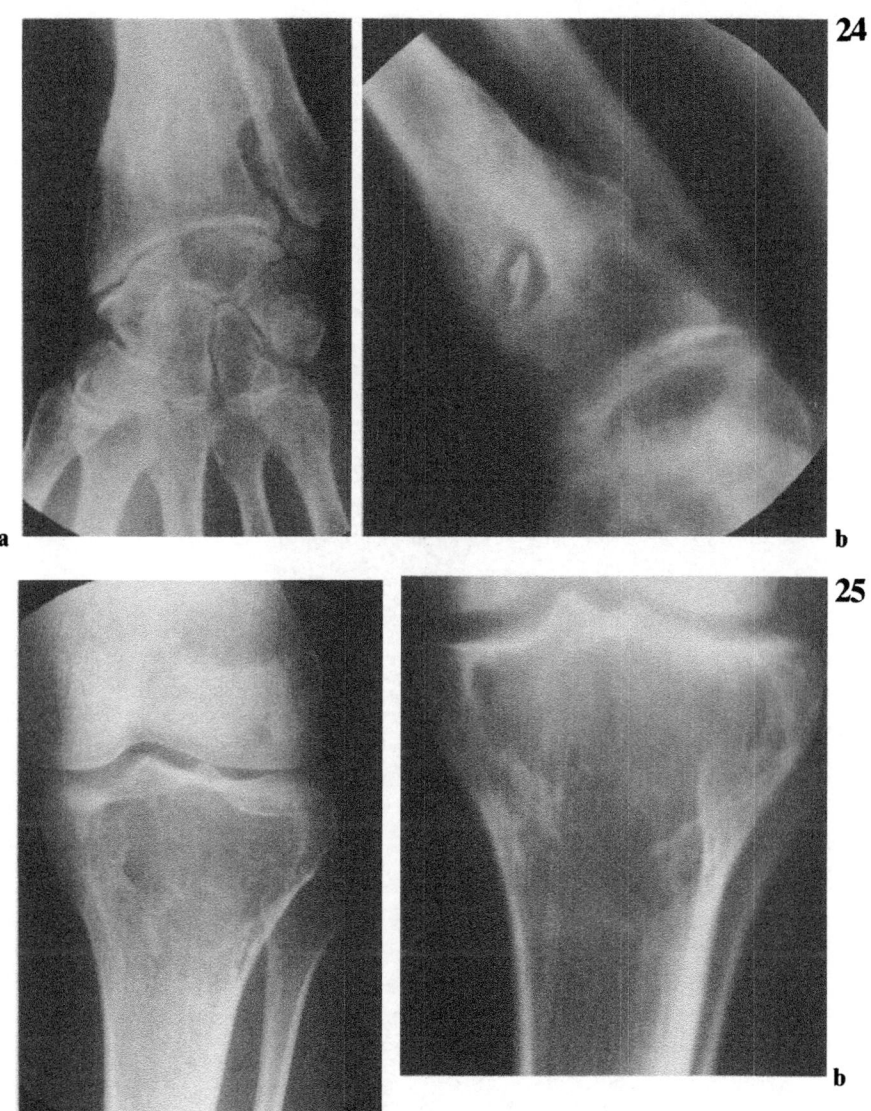

26

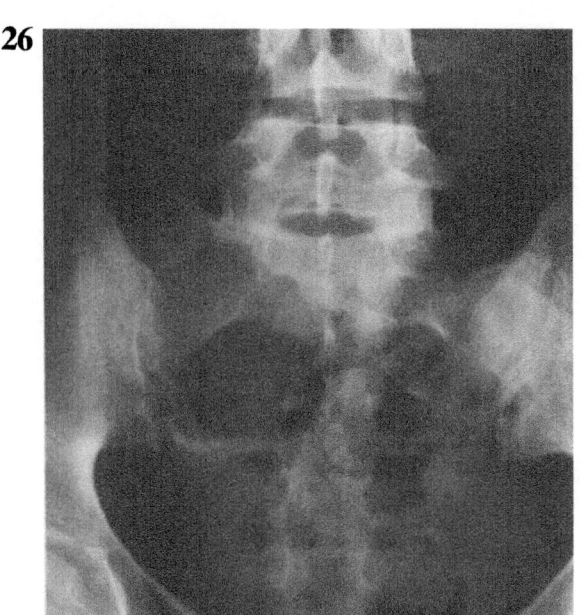

a

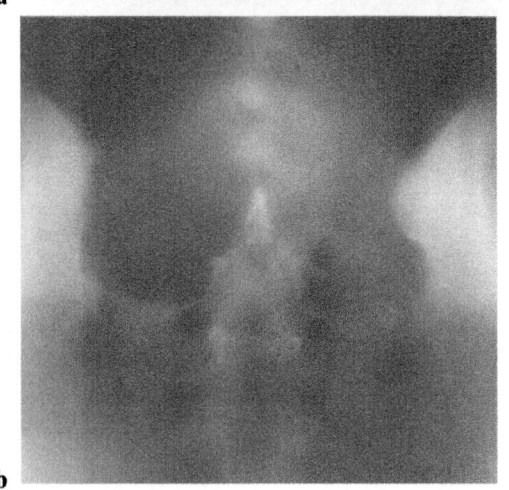

b

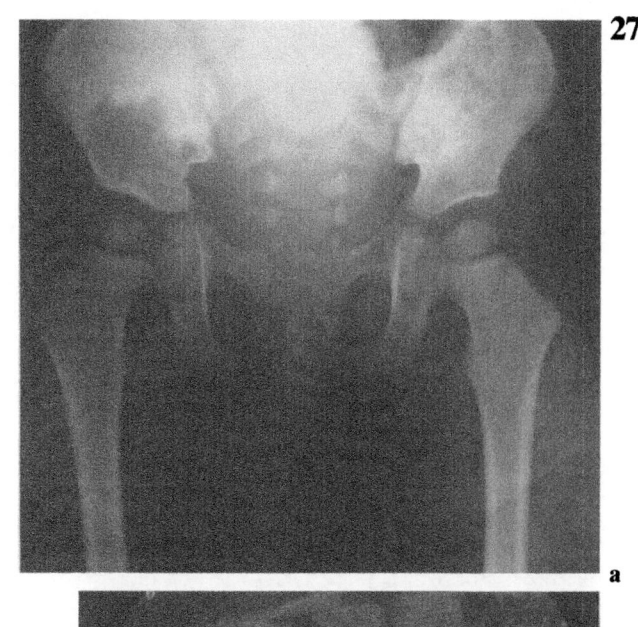

a

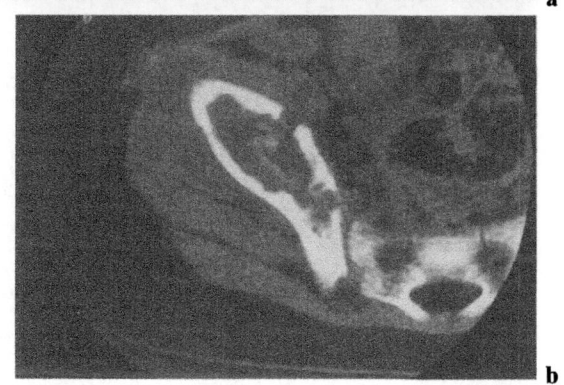

b

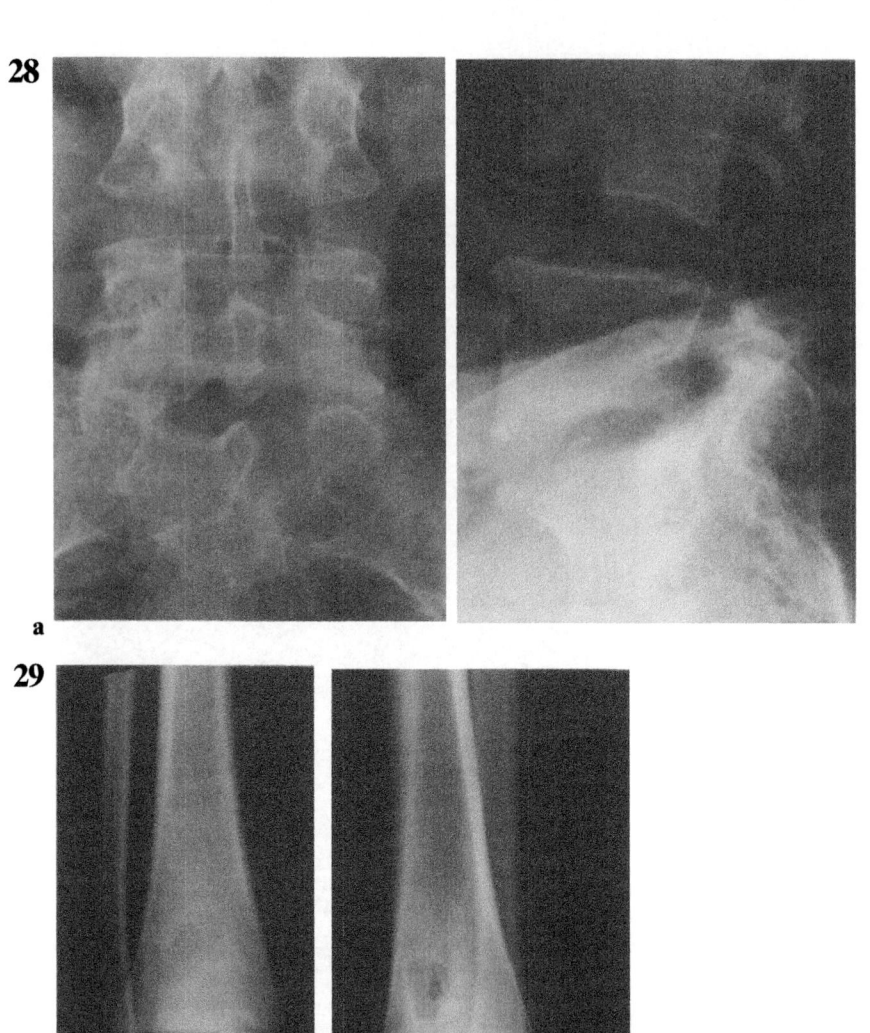

30
32

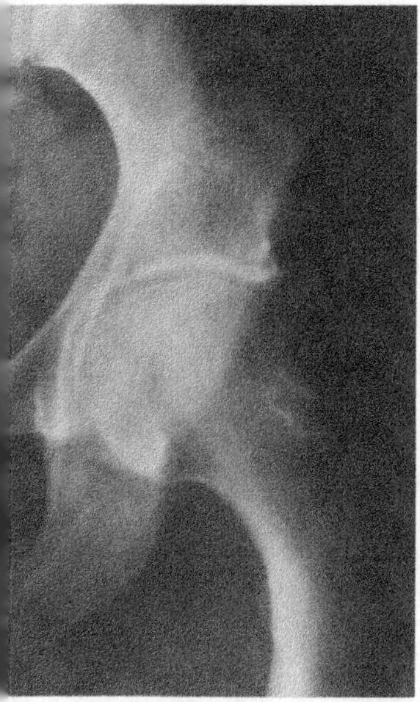

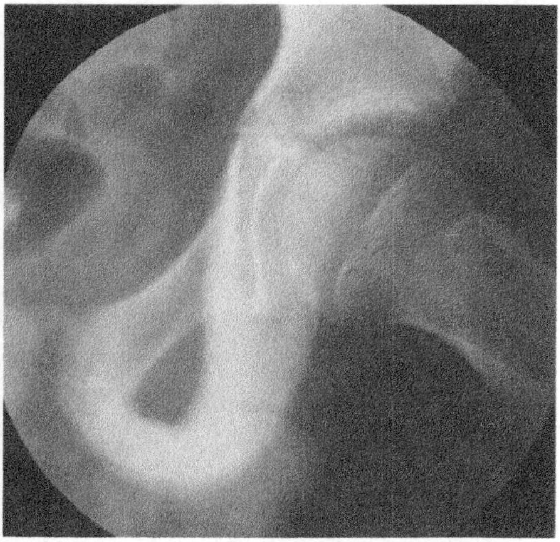

31

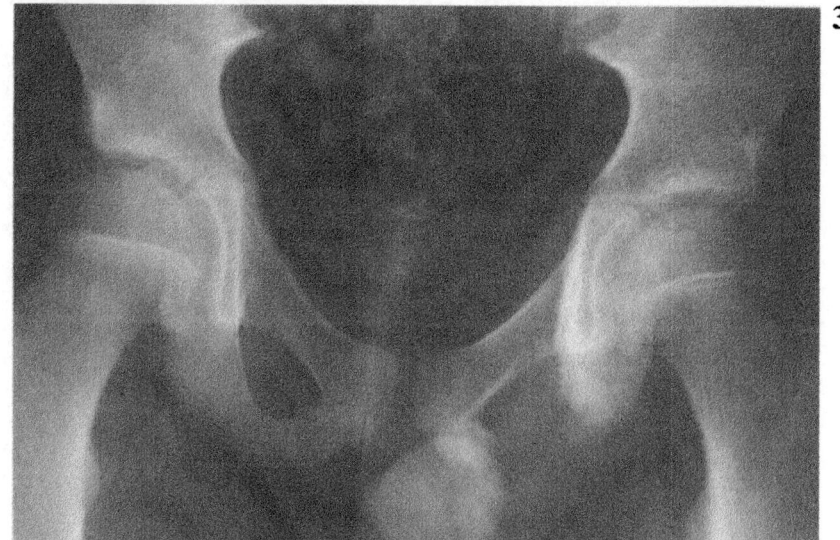

33

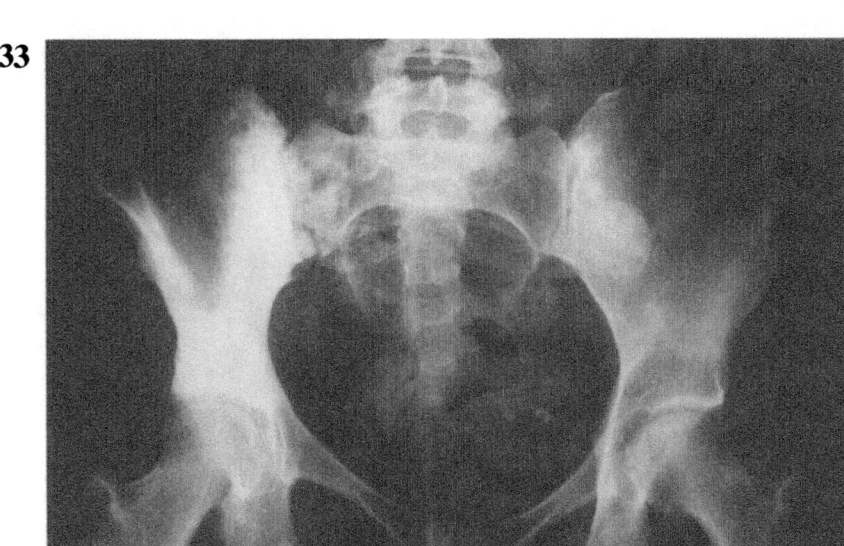

34

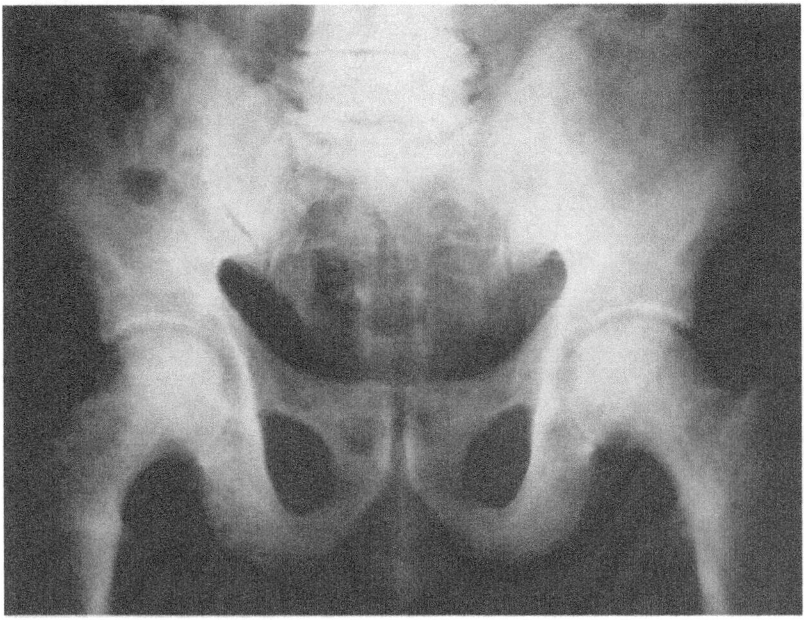

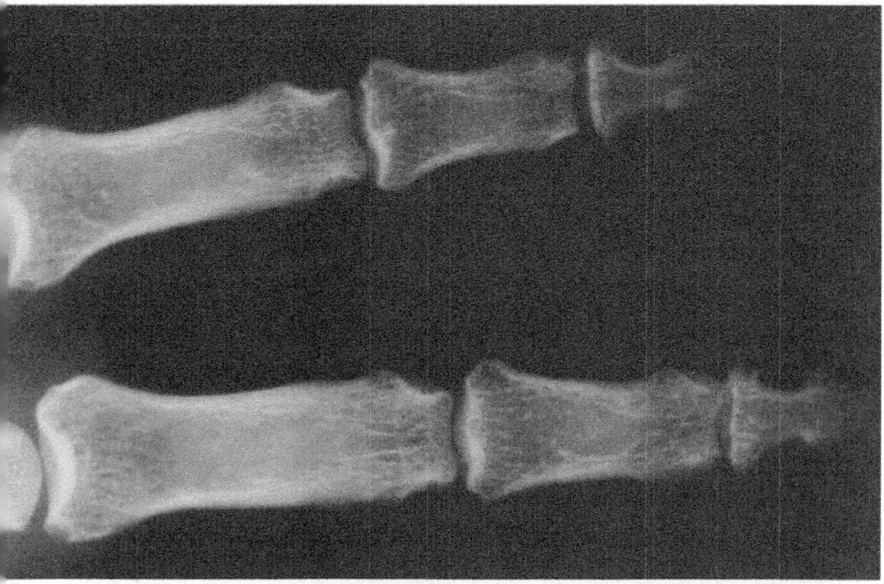

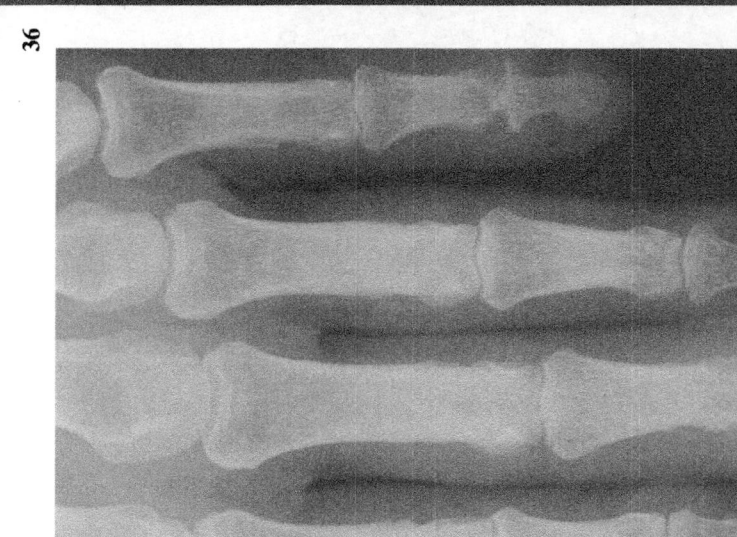

37

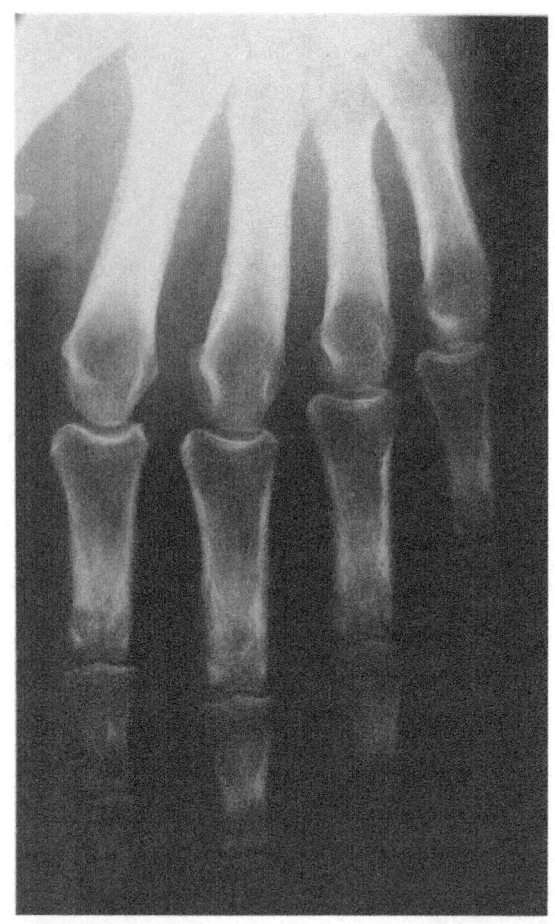

38

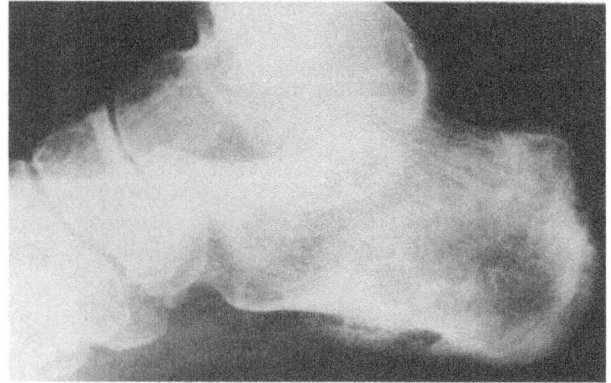

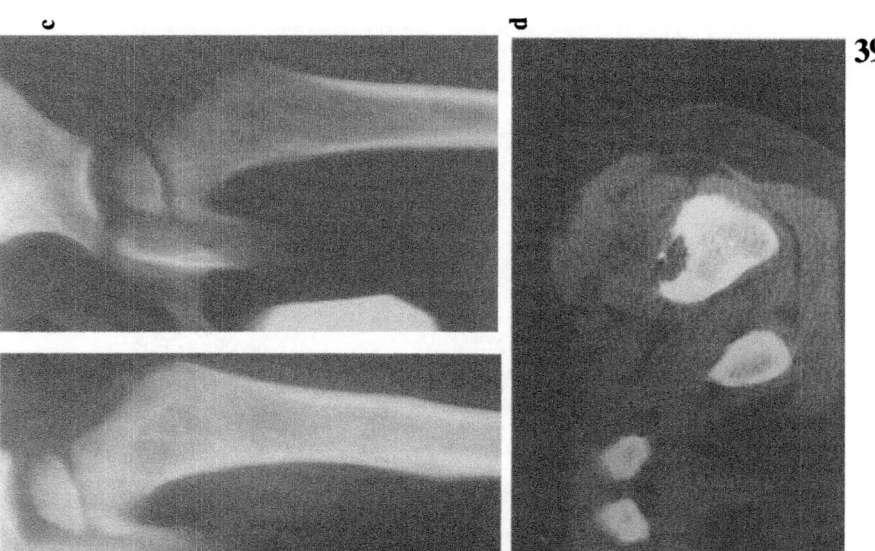

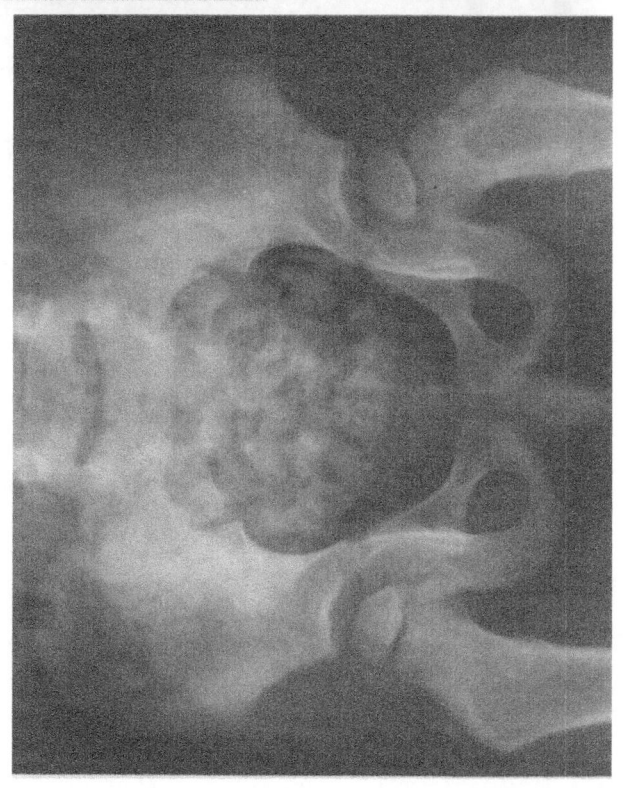

39

27

40-
43

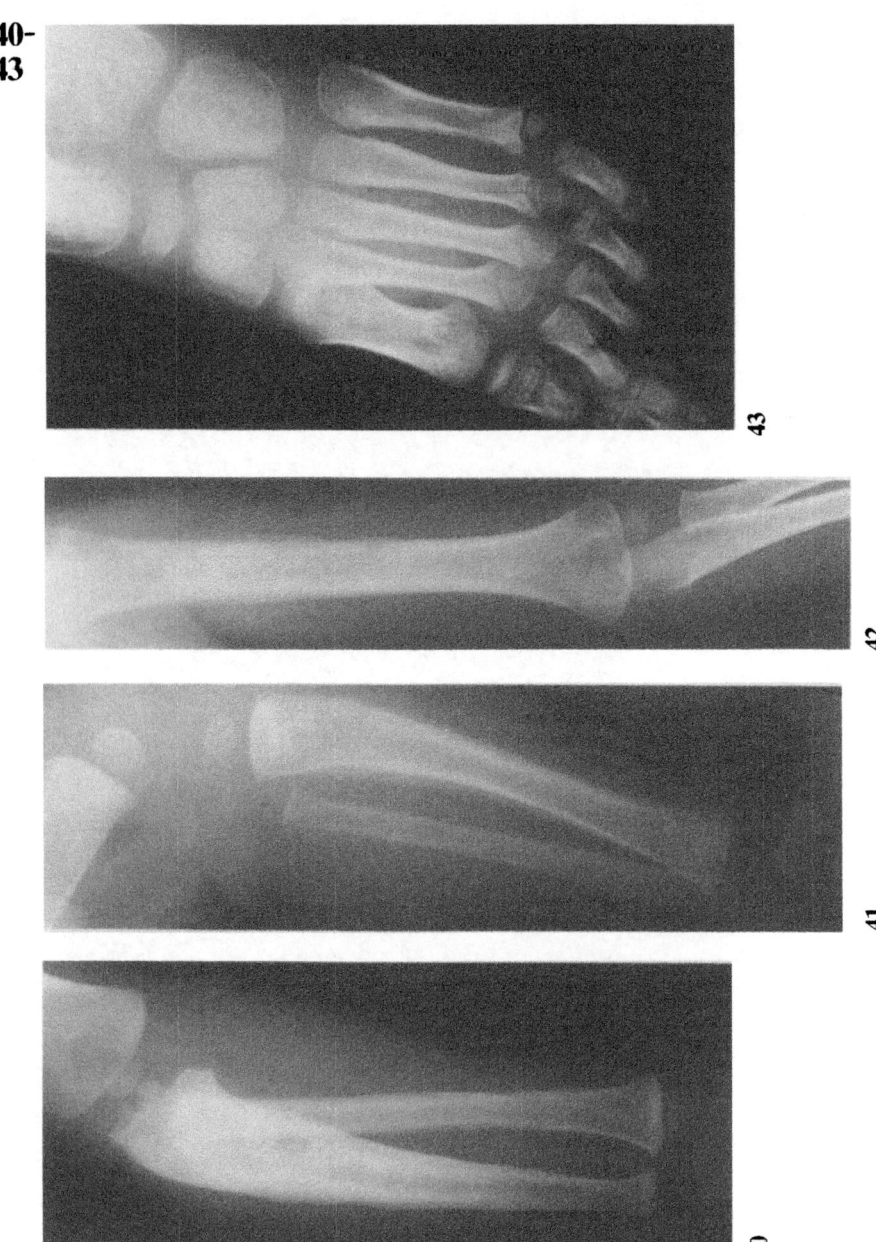

43

42

41

40

28

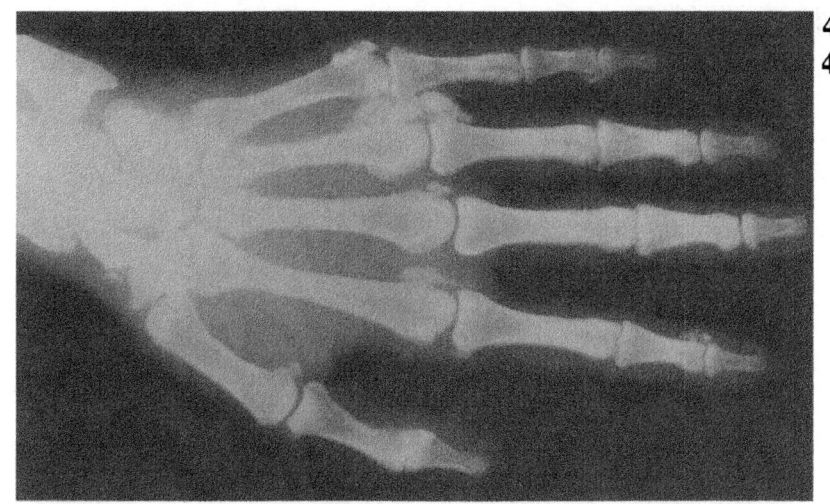

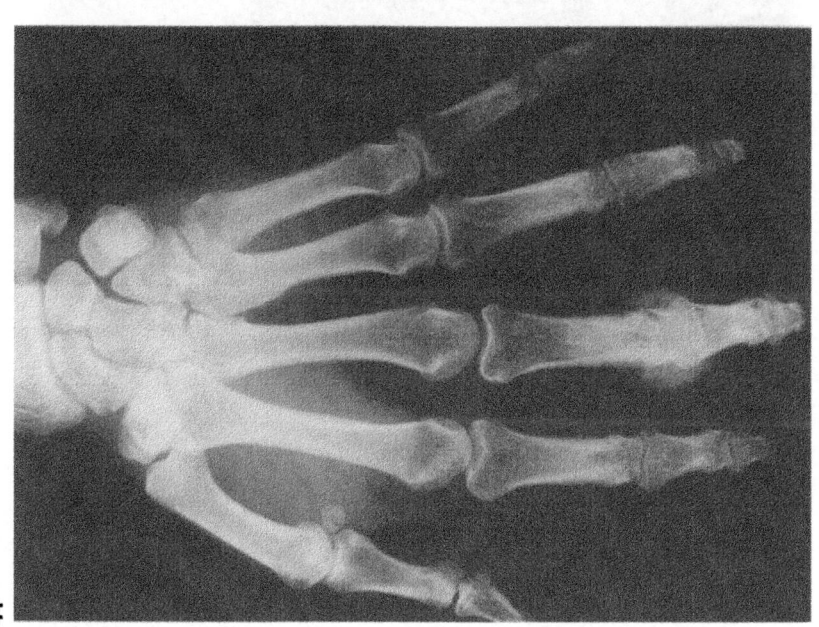

46

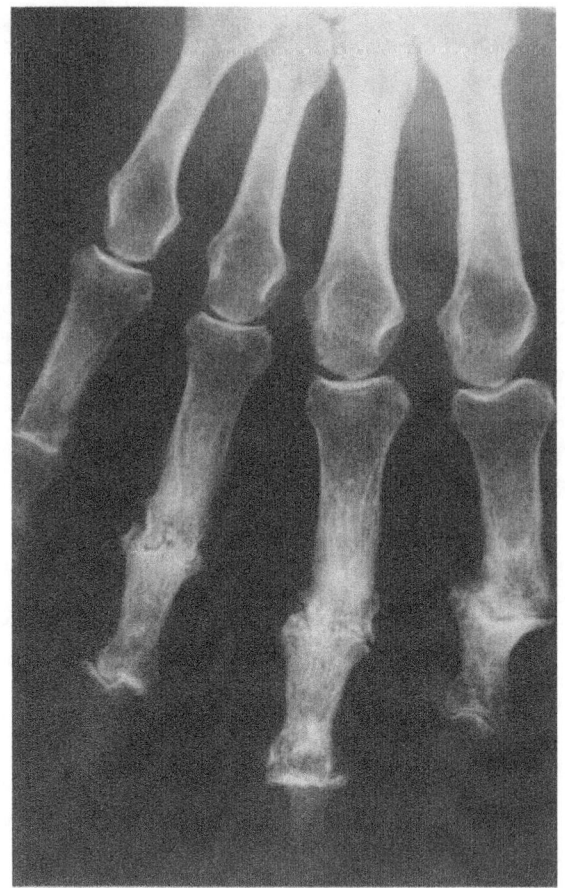

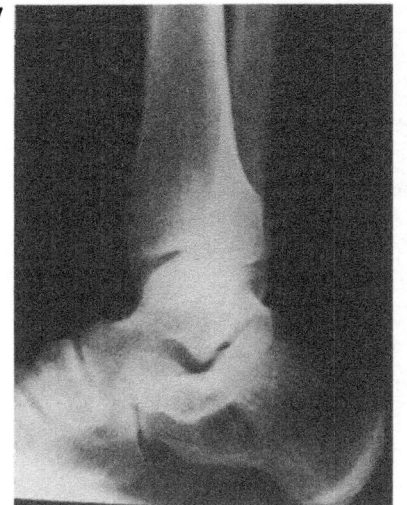

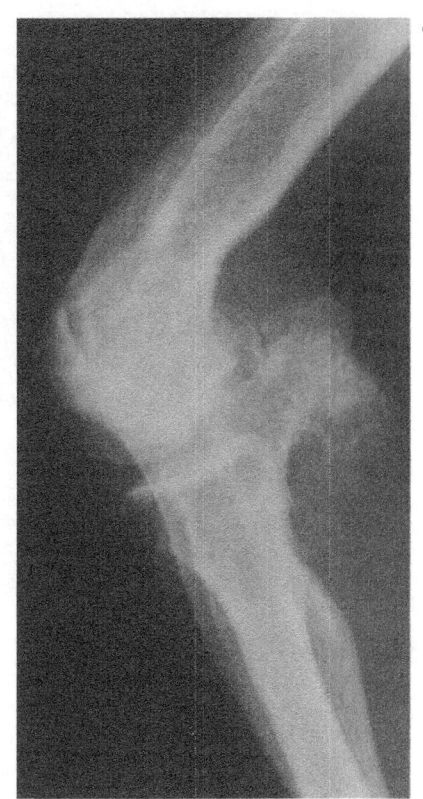

49

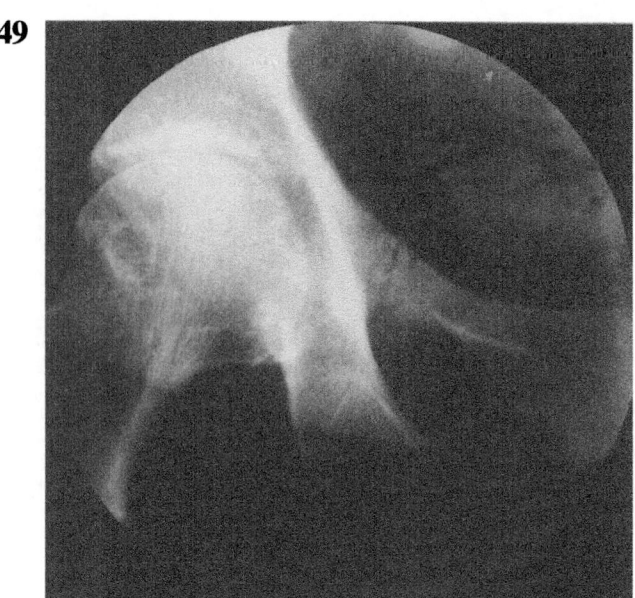

50

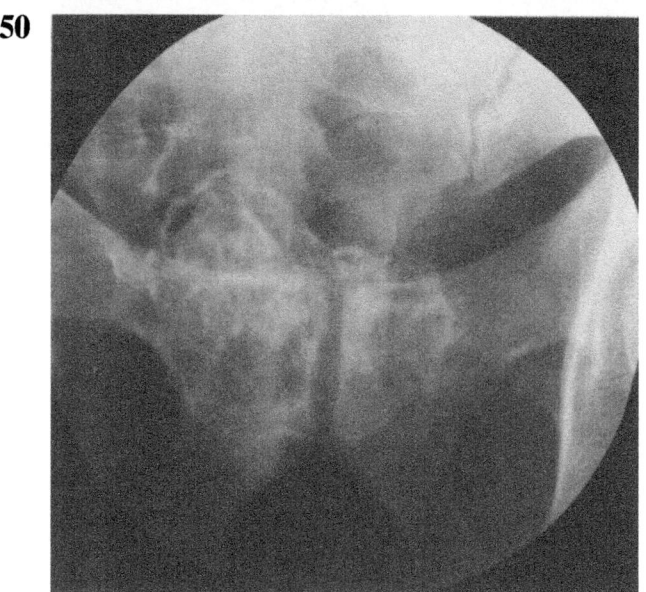

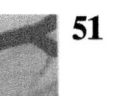
51

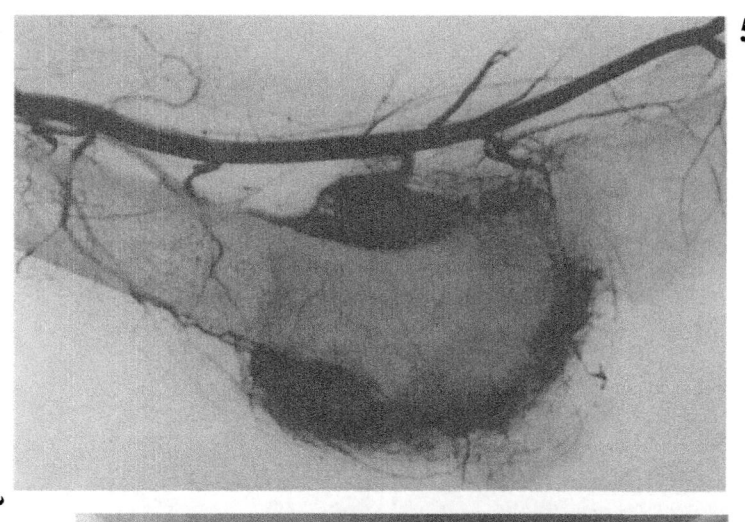

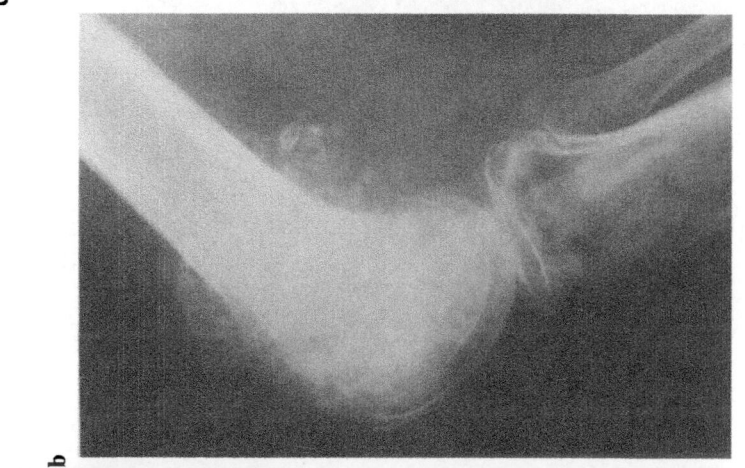

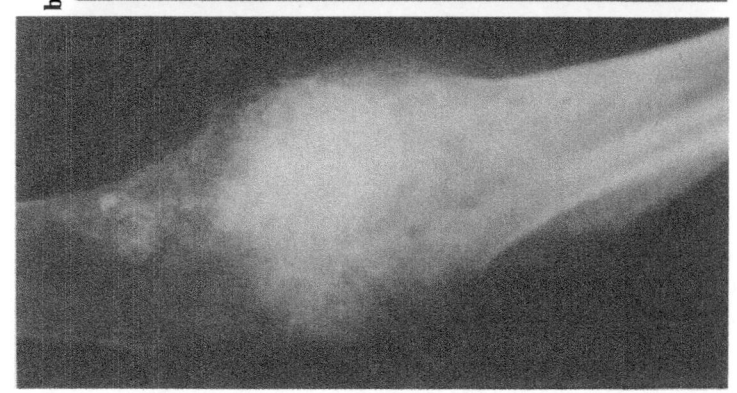

52

a

b

c

34

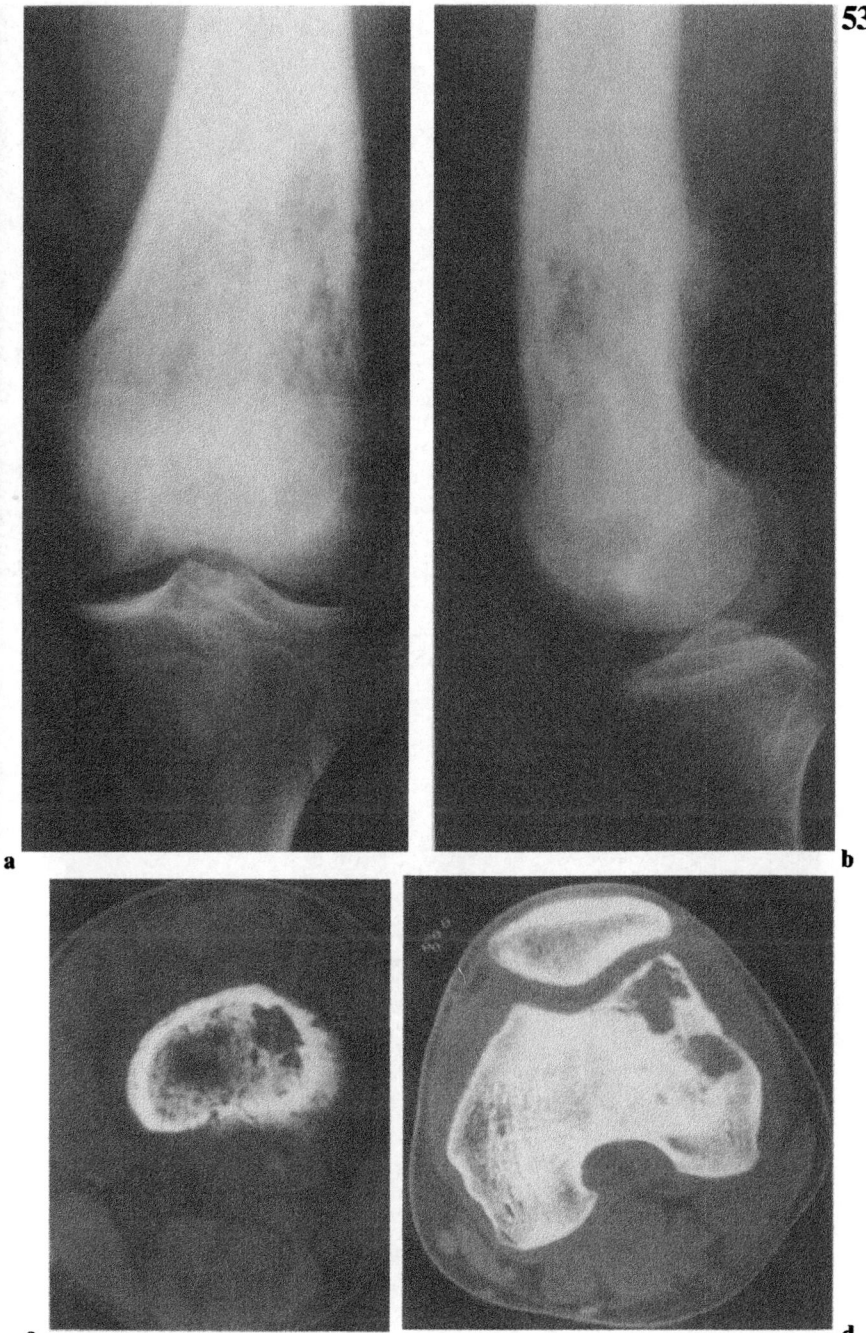

a

b

c

d

54

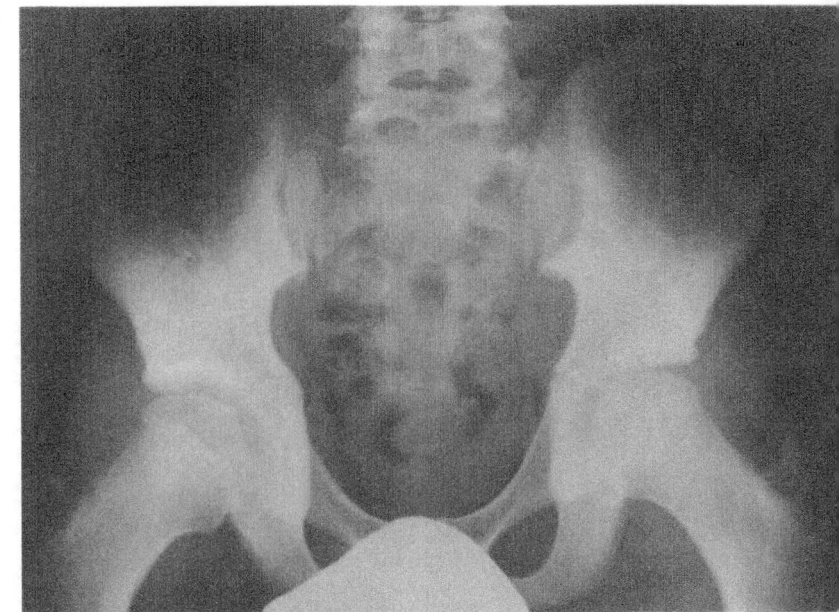

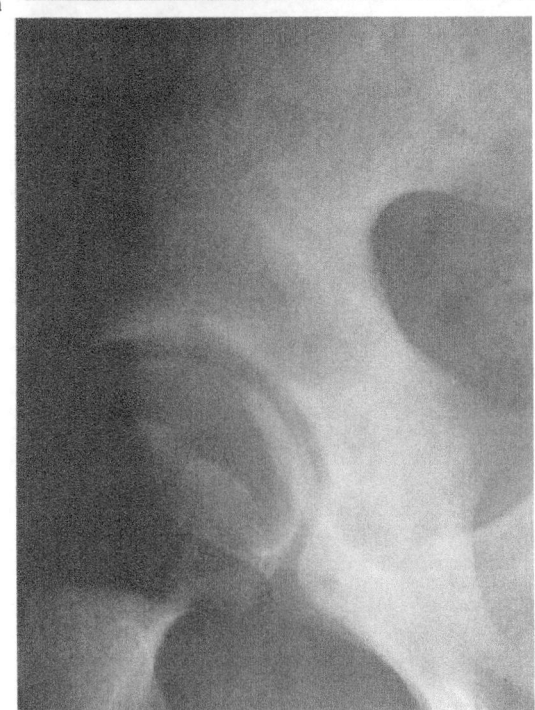

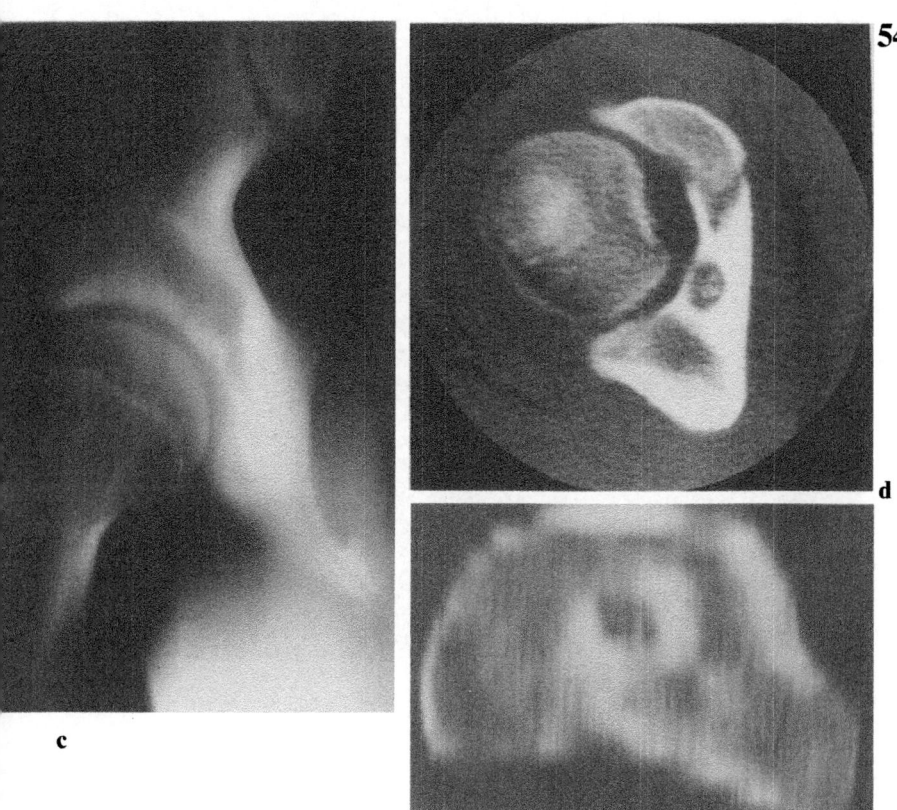

c

d

e

55

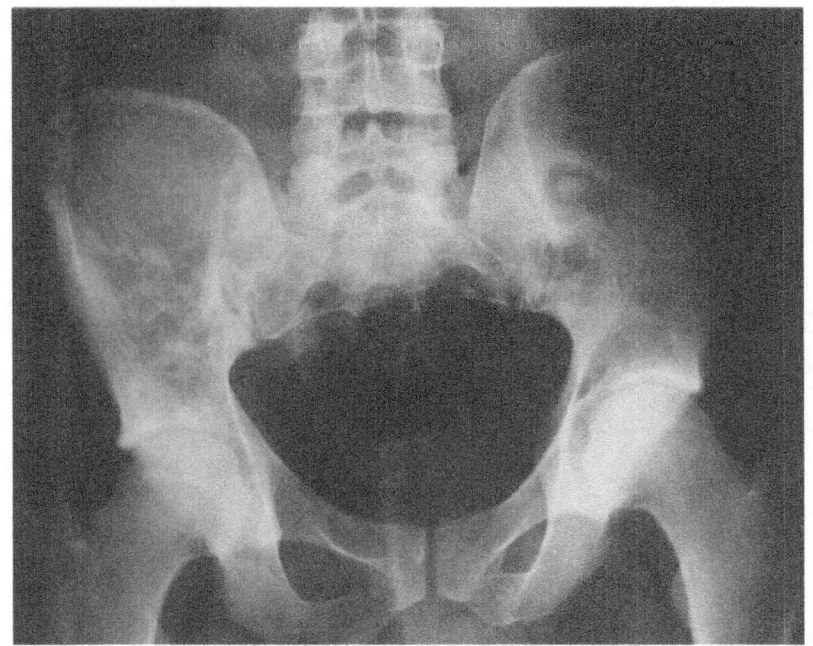

a

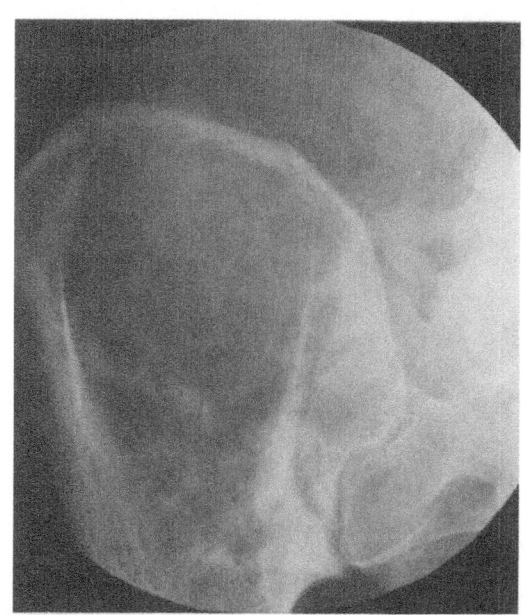

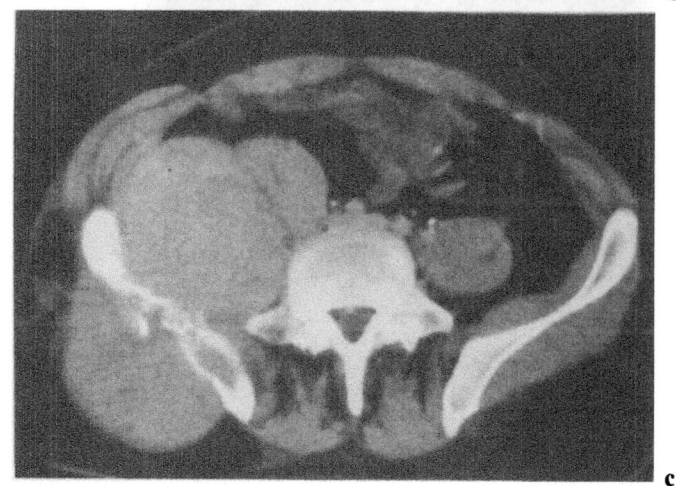

56

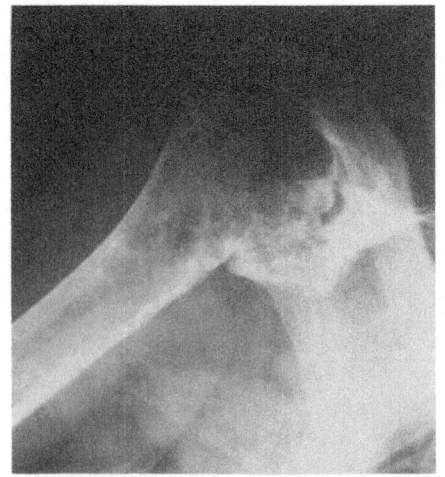

57

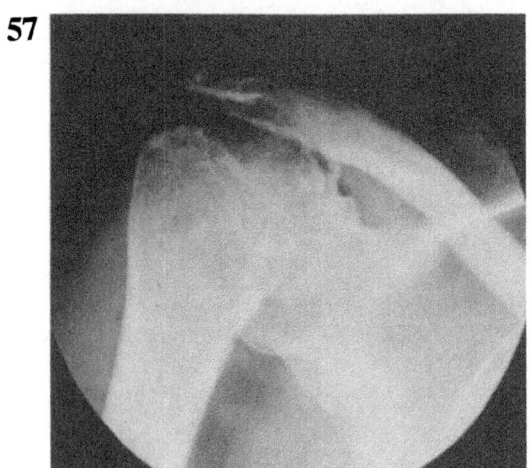

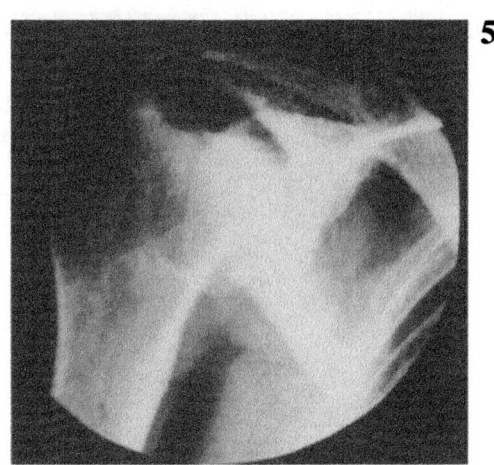

58

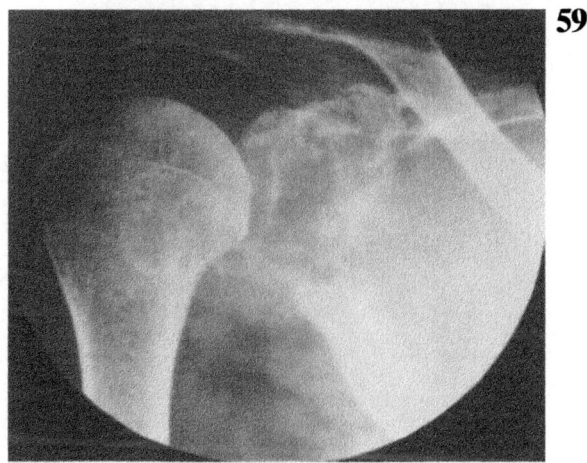

59

60

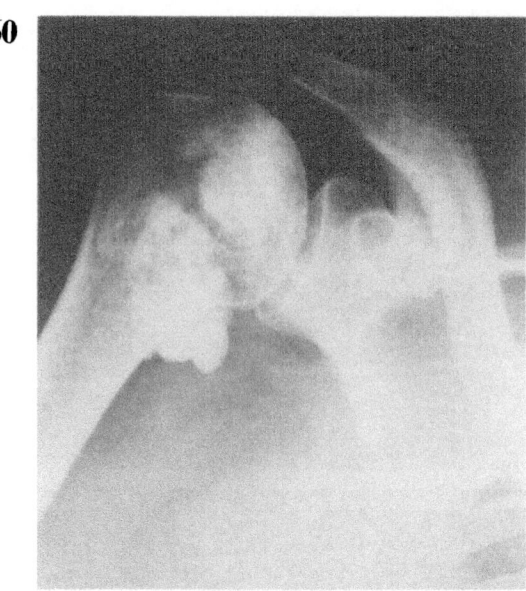

61

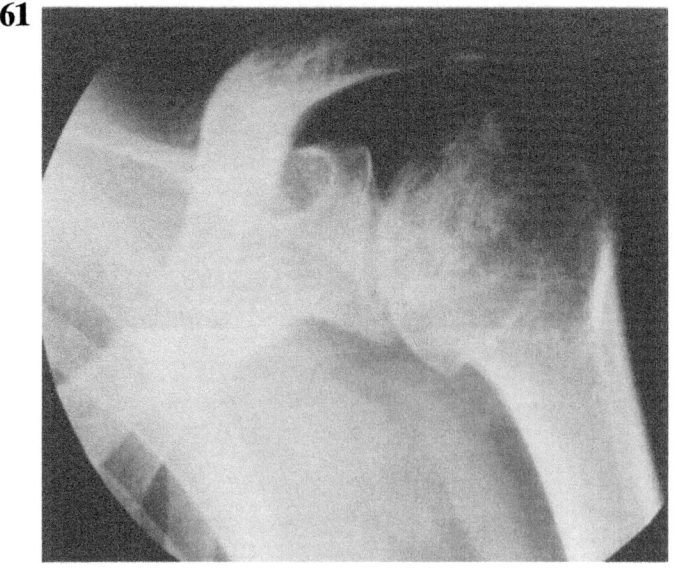

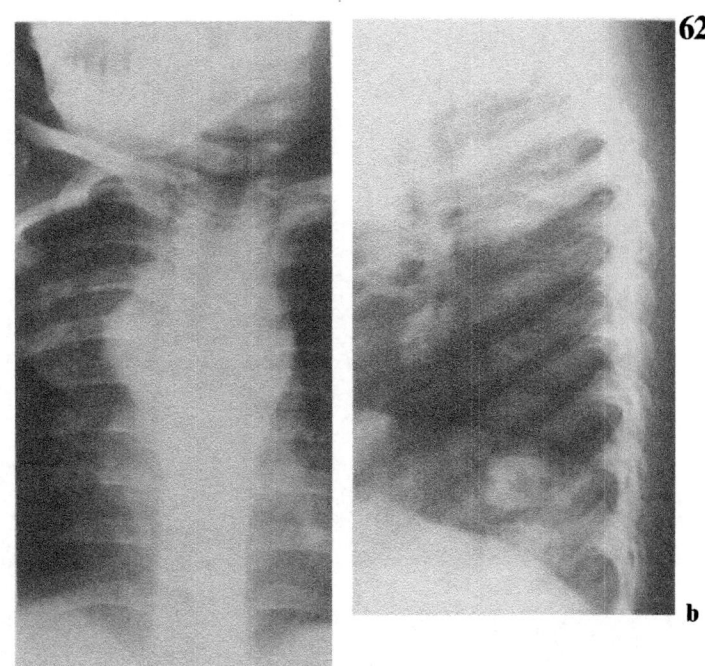

a

b

63

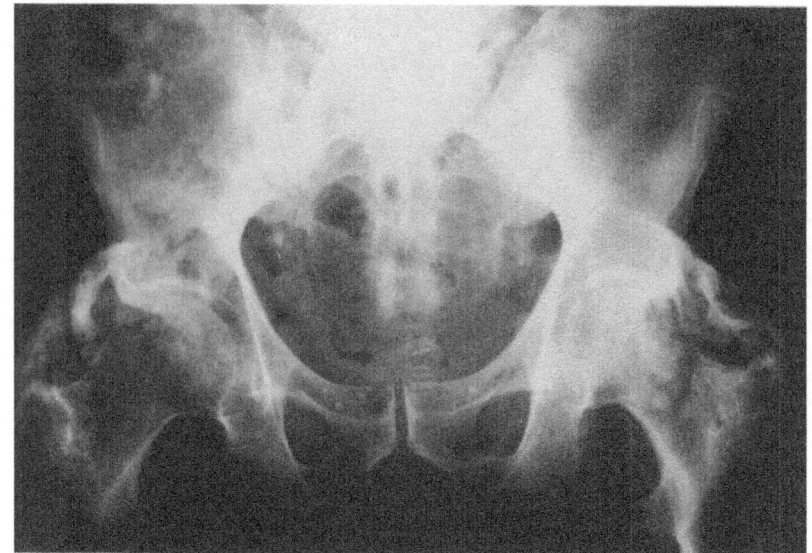

64

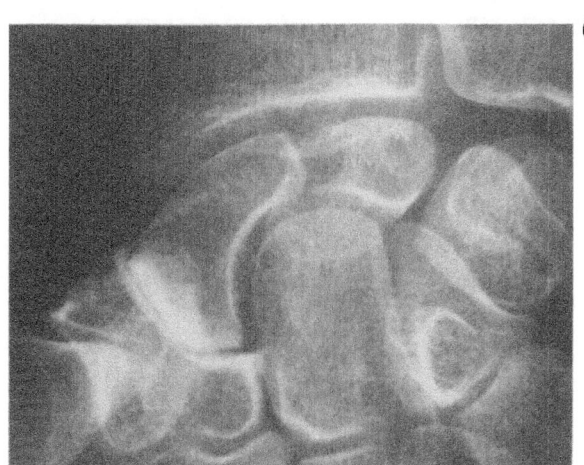

65

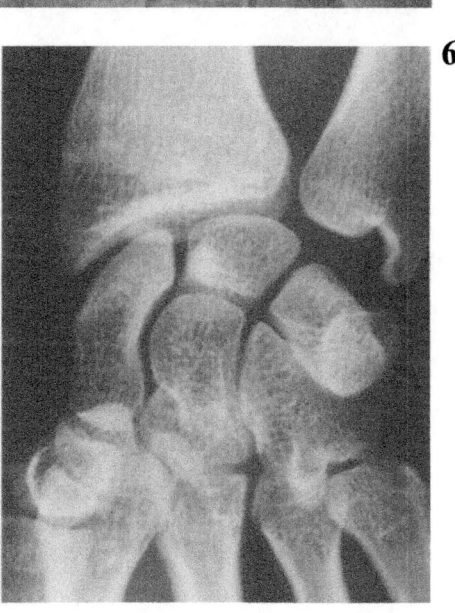

66

67

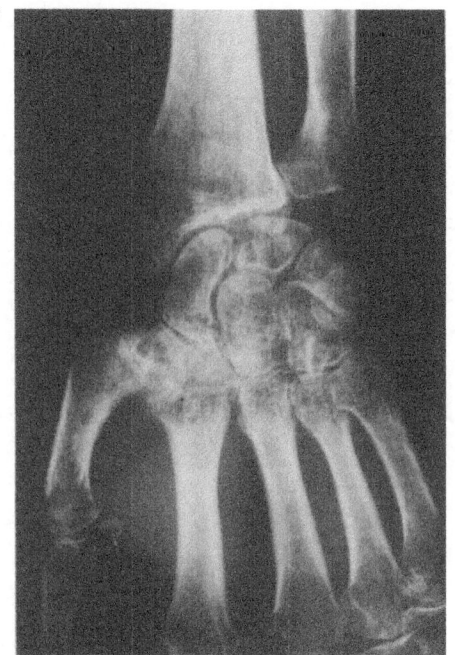

68

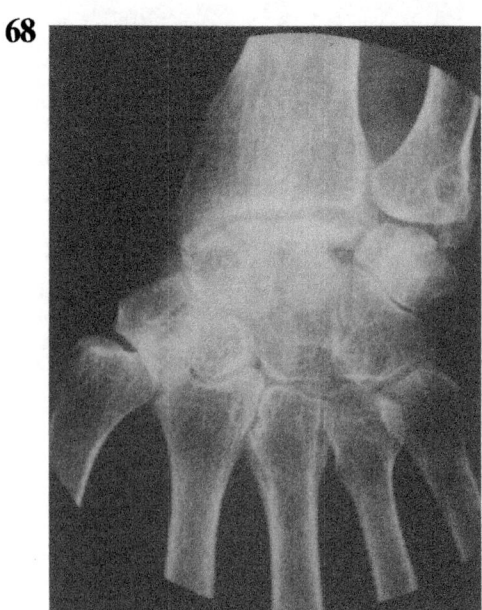

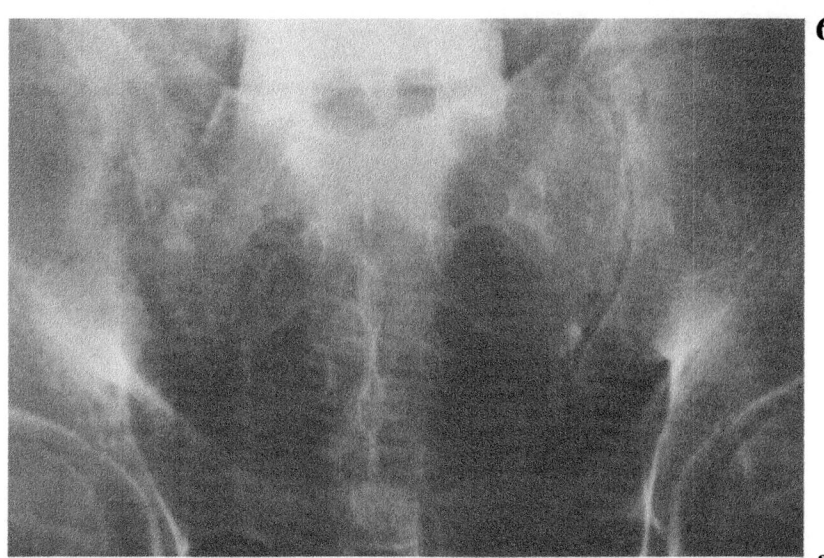

a

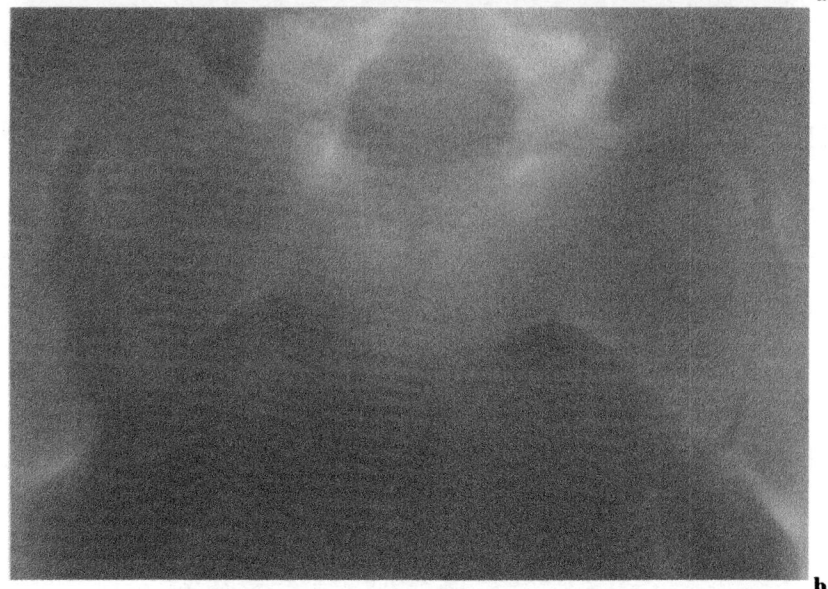

b

70

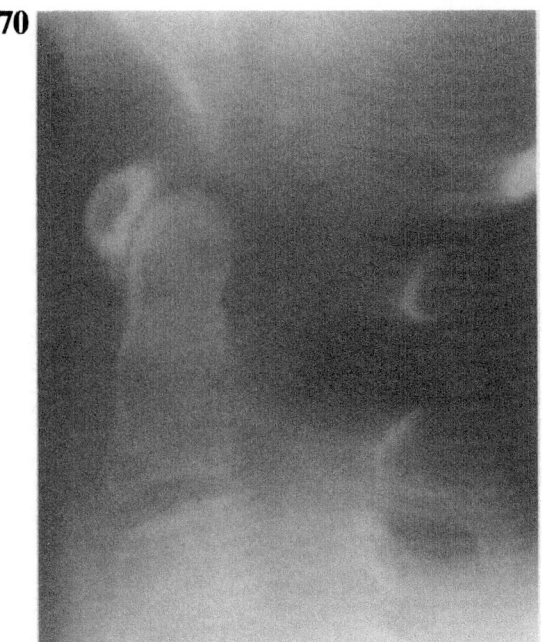

71

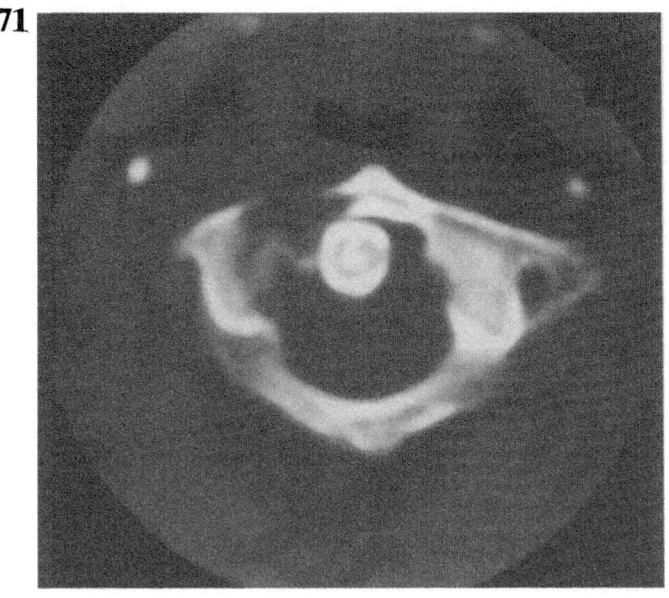

72

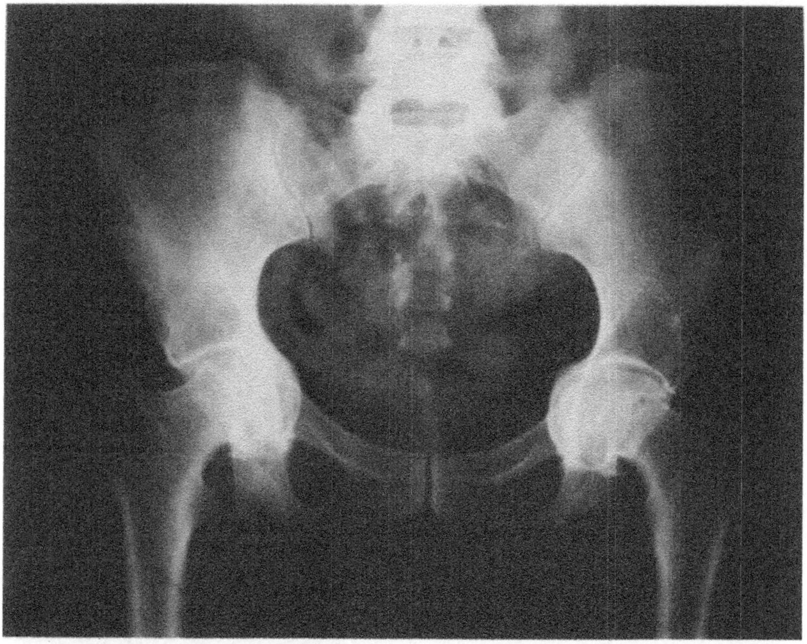

73

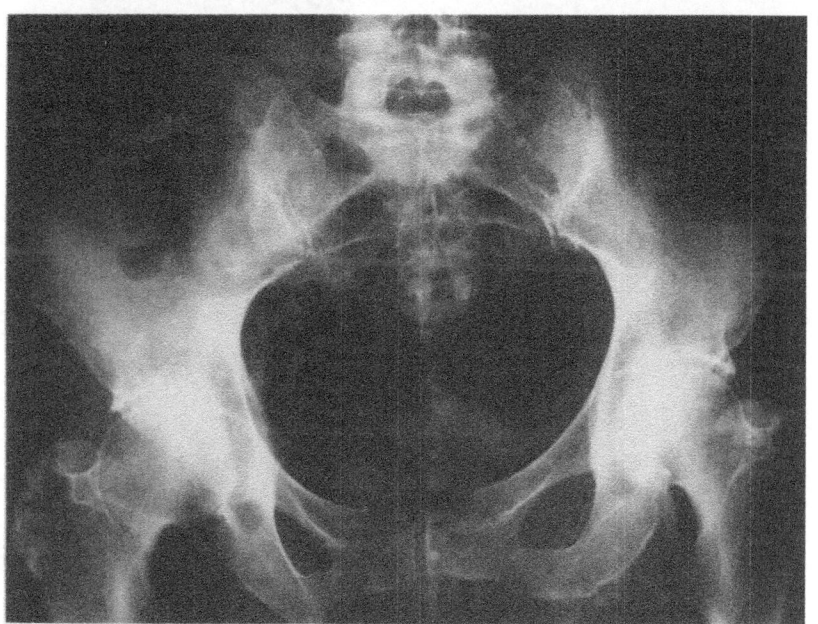

74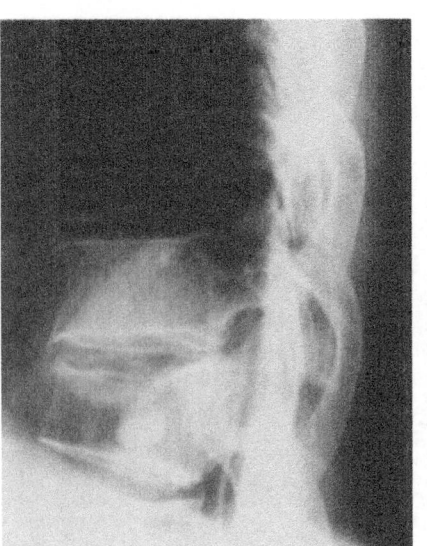

75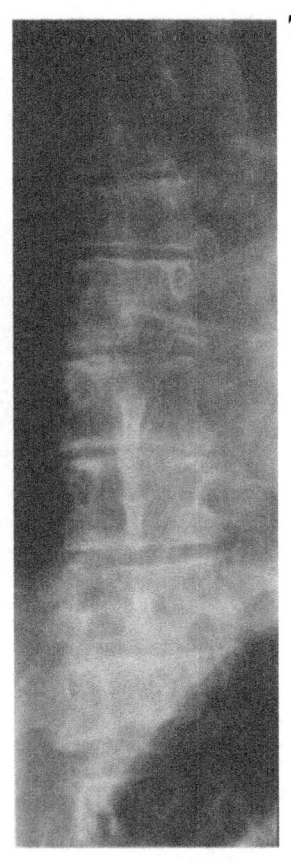

76

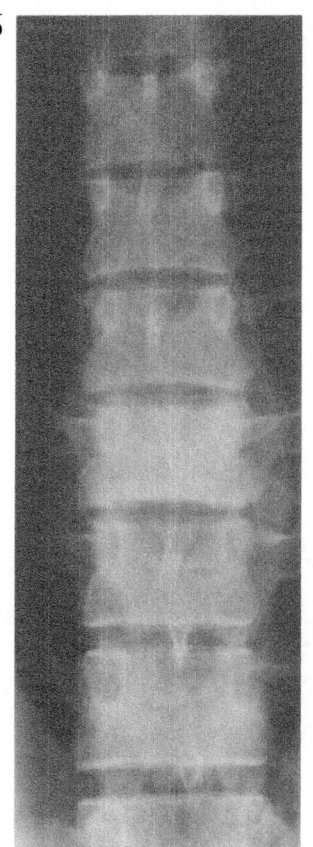

77

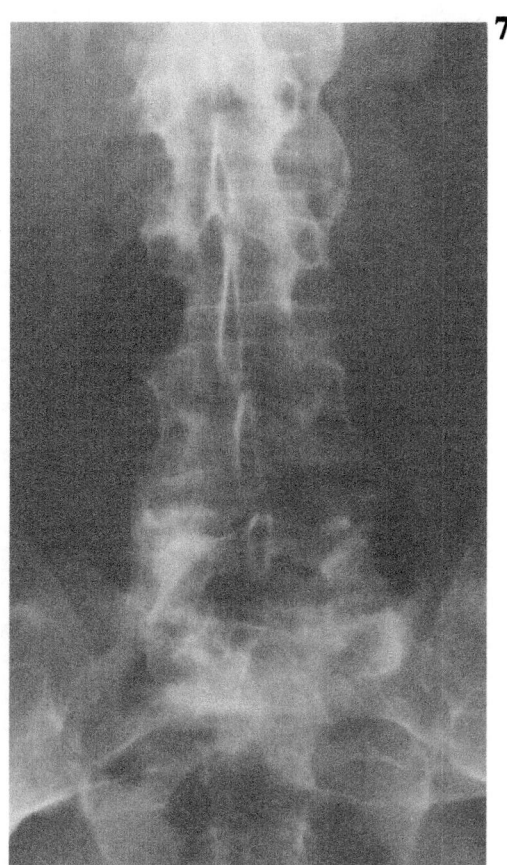

78
79

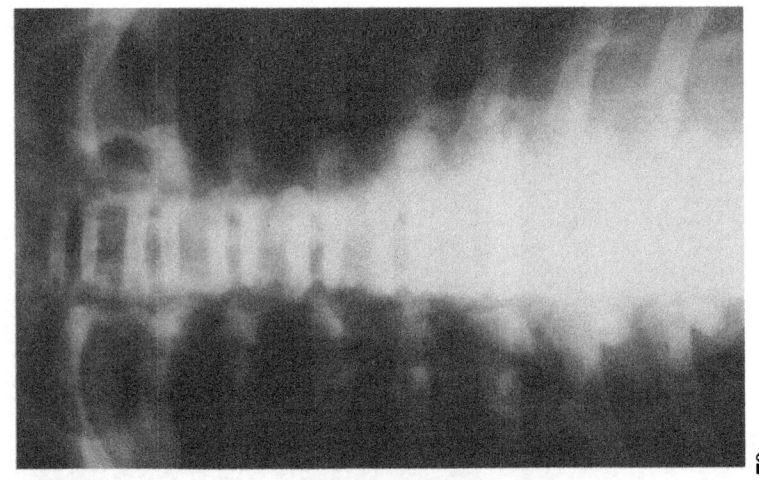

79

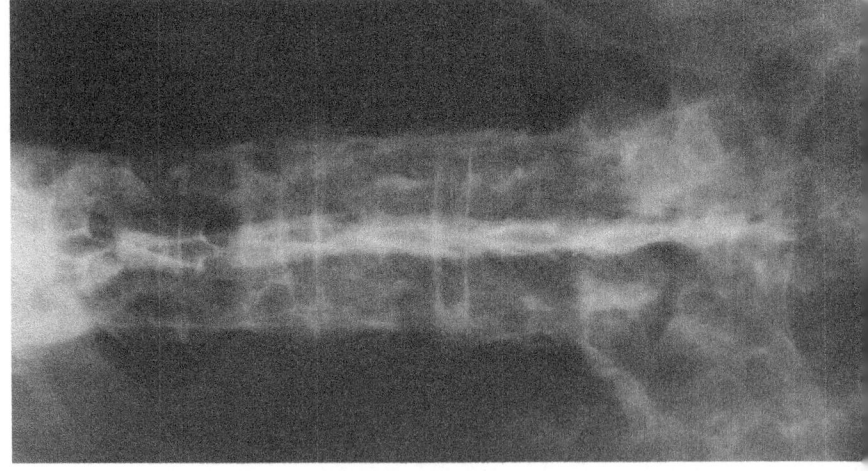

78

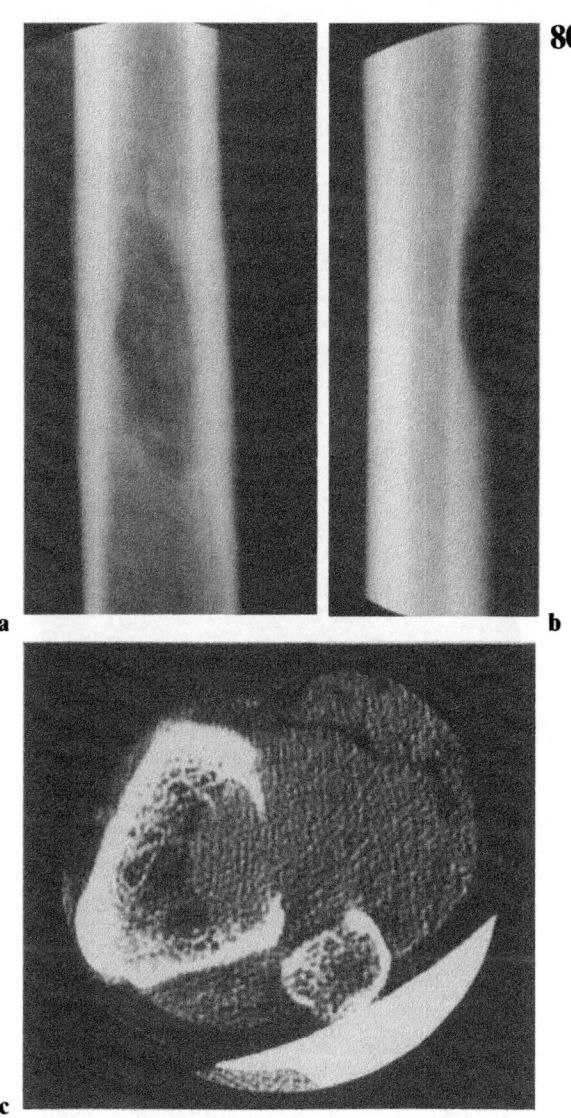

80

a

b

c

81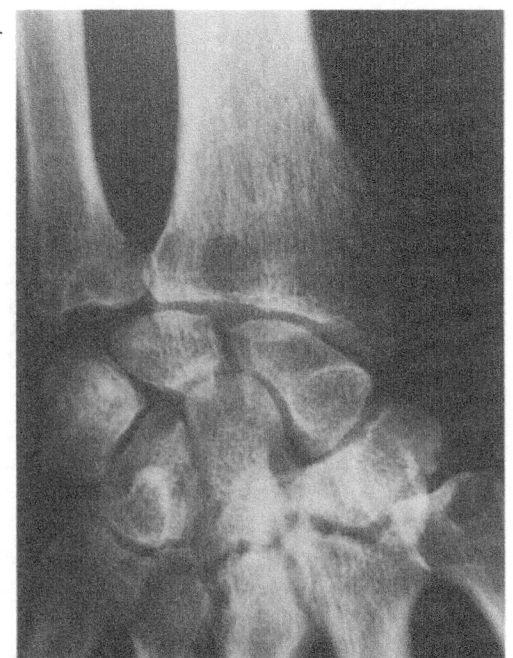

82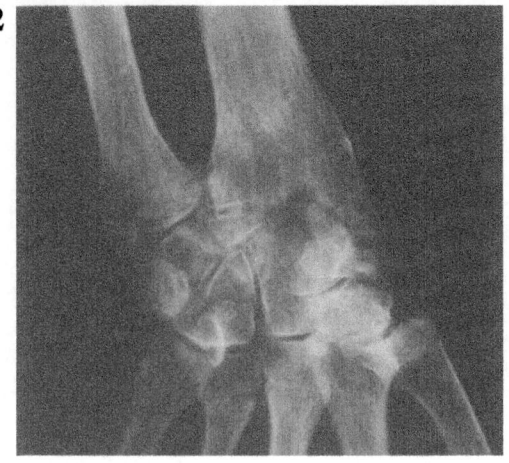

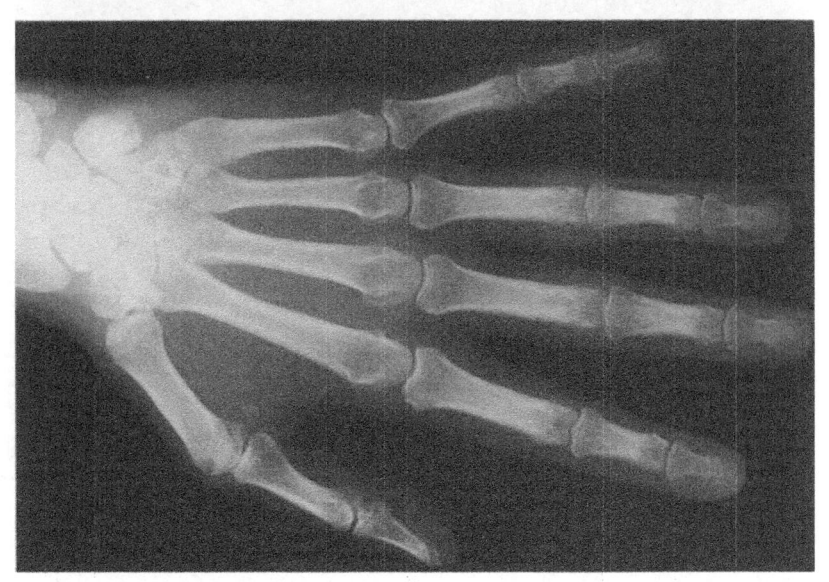

83
84

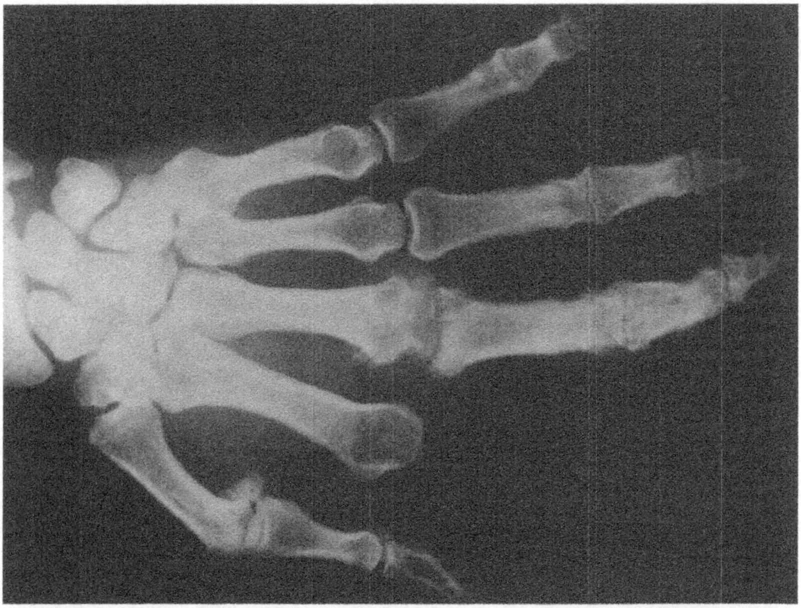

84

83

55

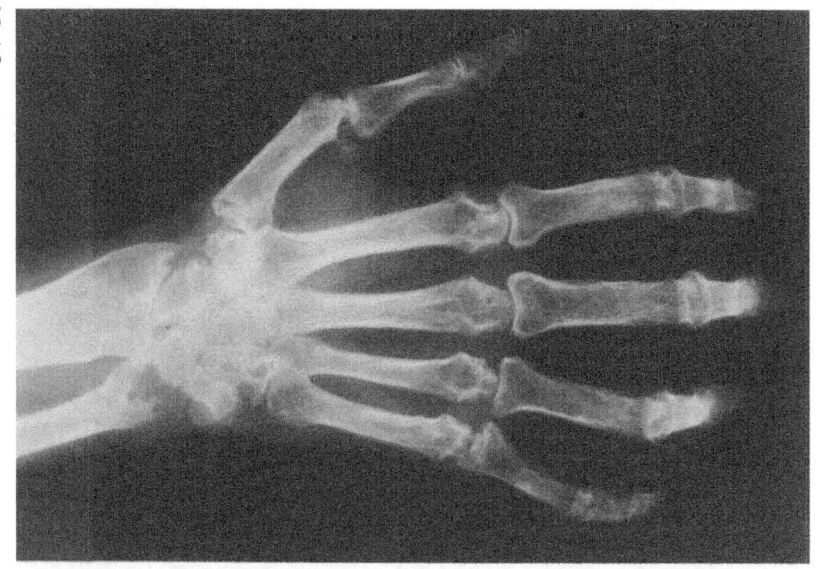

86

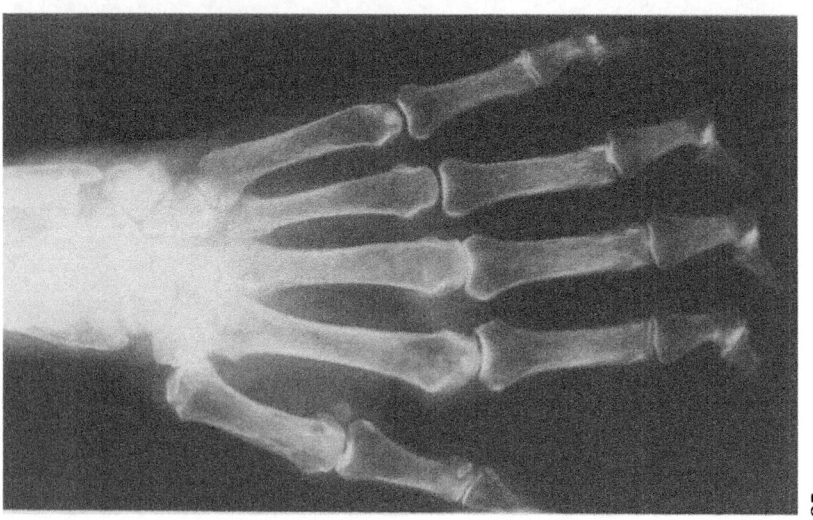

85

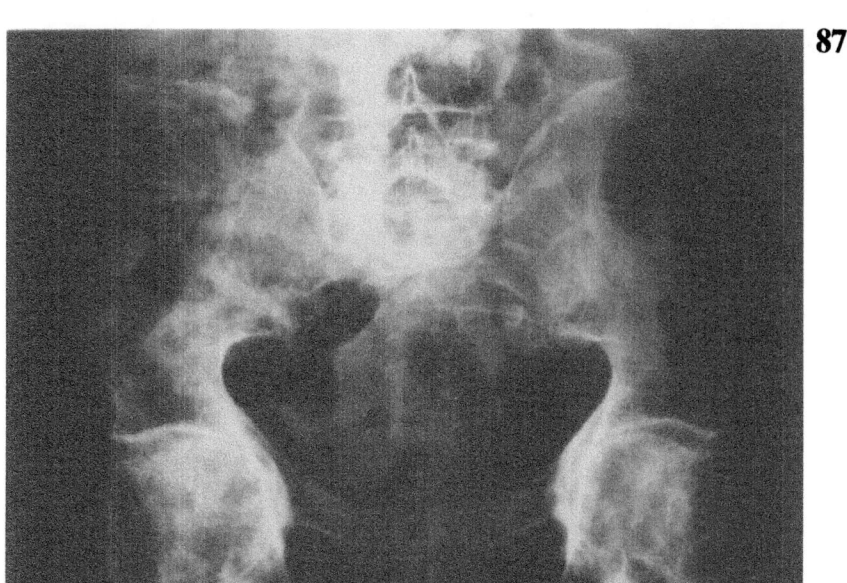

87

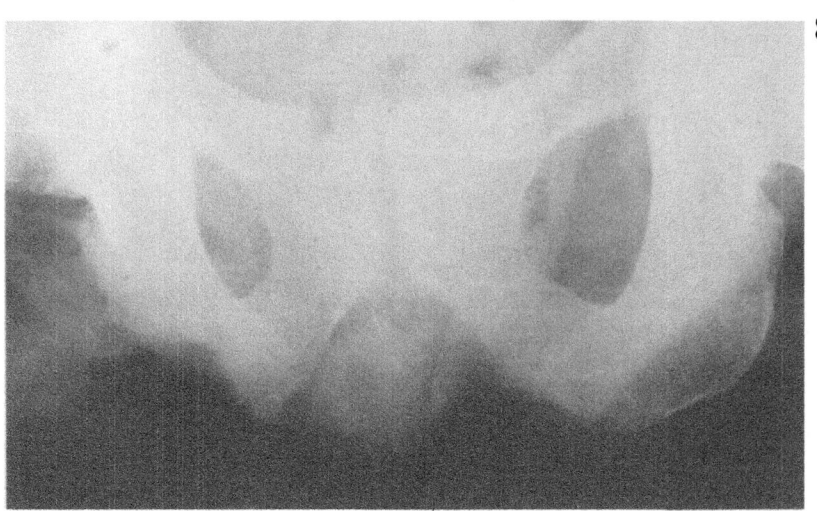

88

89
90

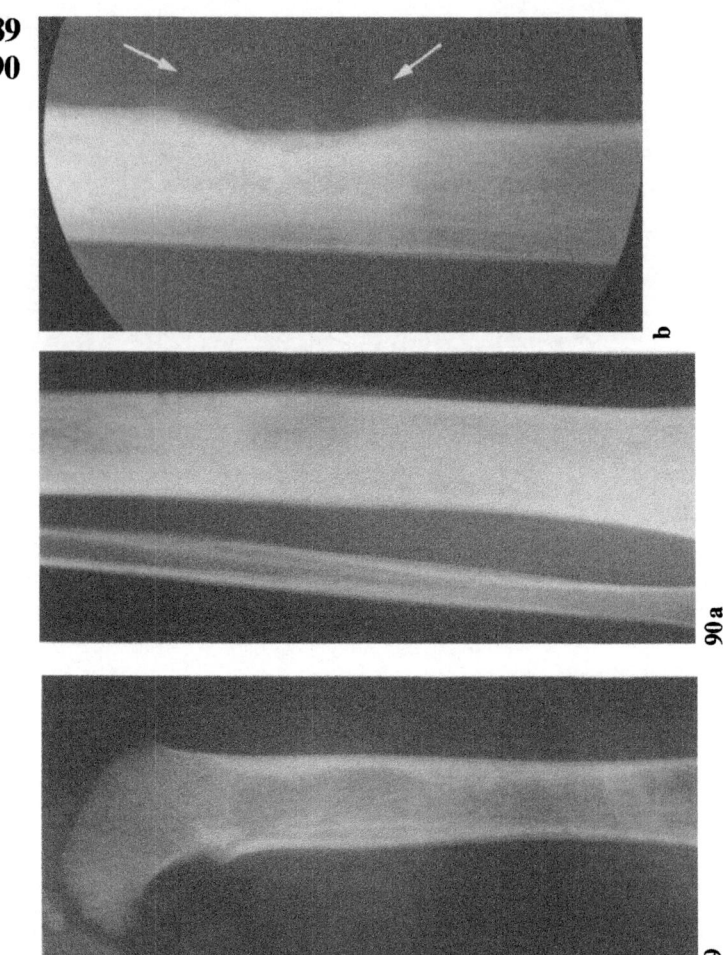

b

90 a

89

58

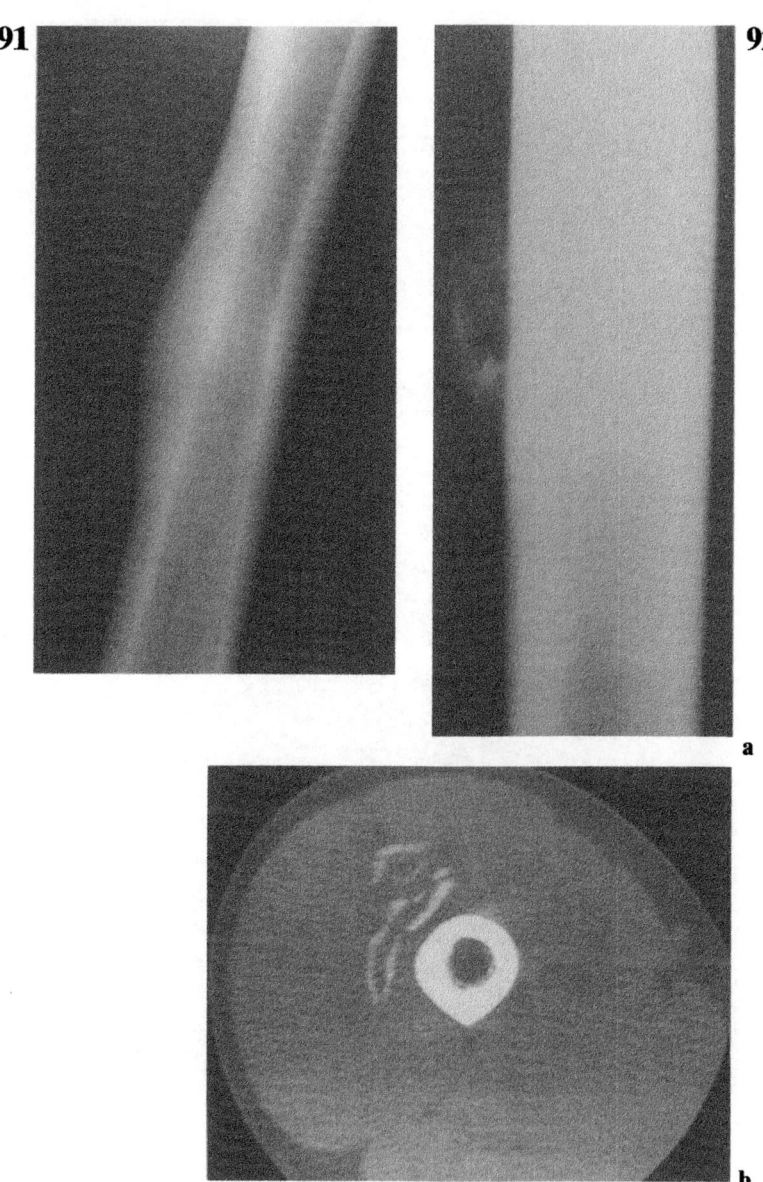

93
94

94

b

93 a

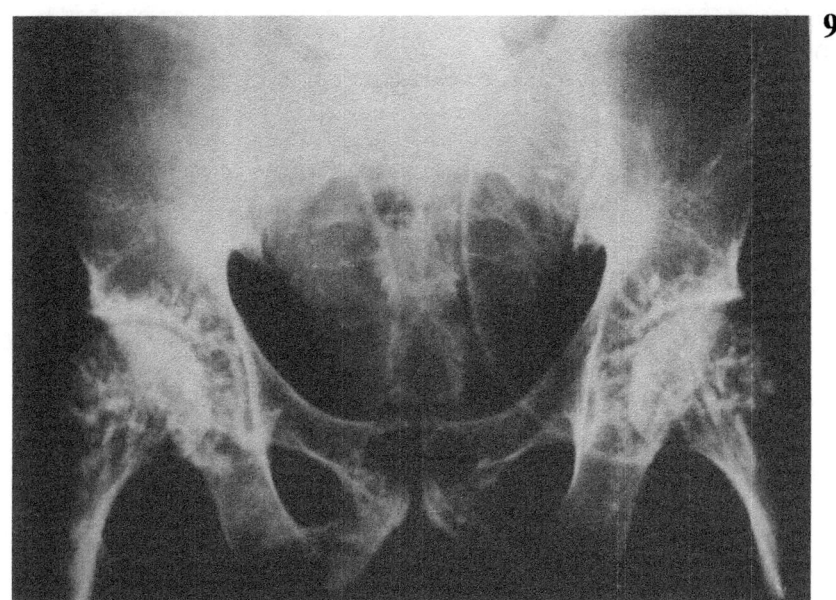

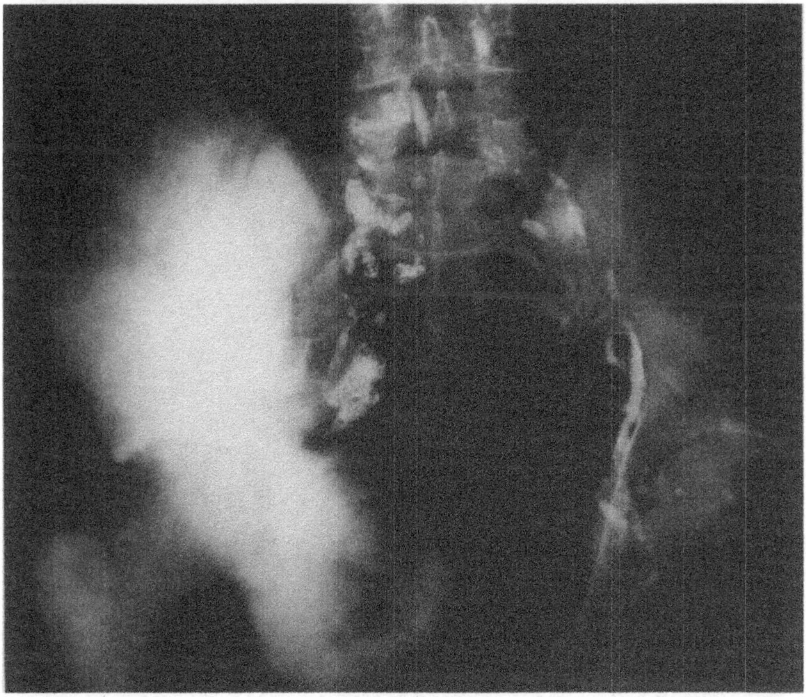

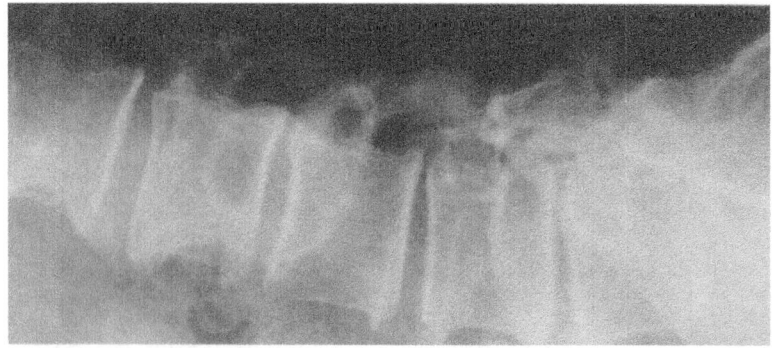

99

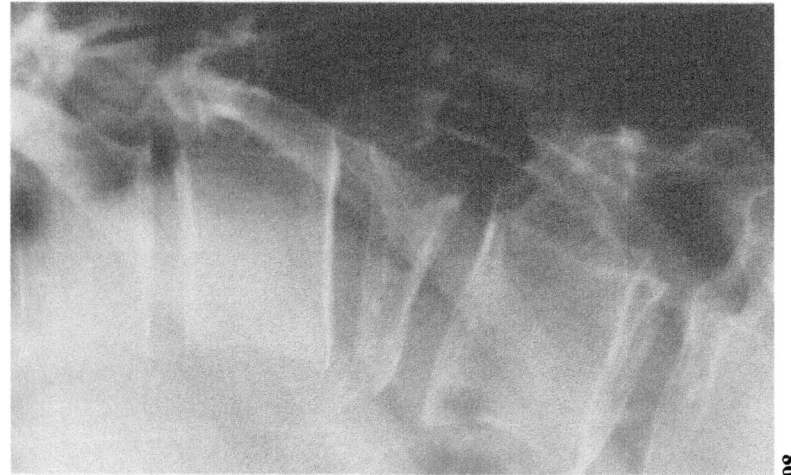

98

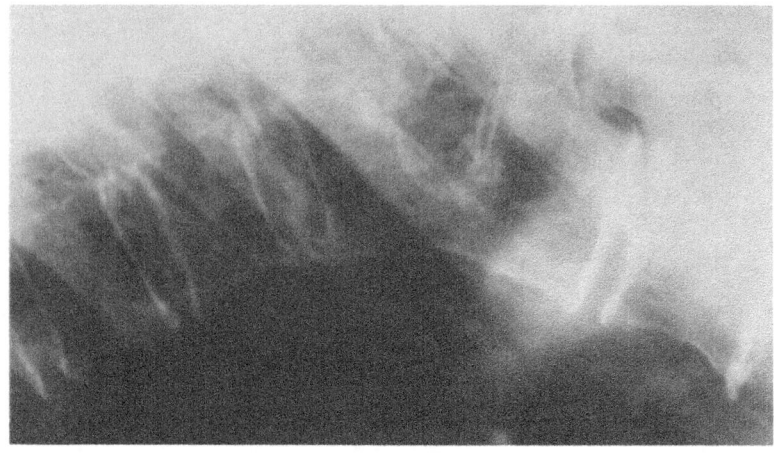

97

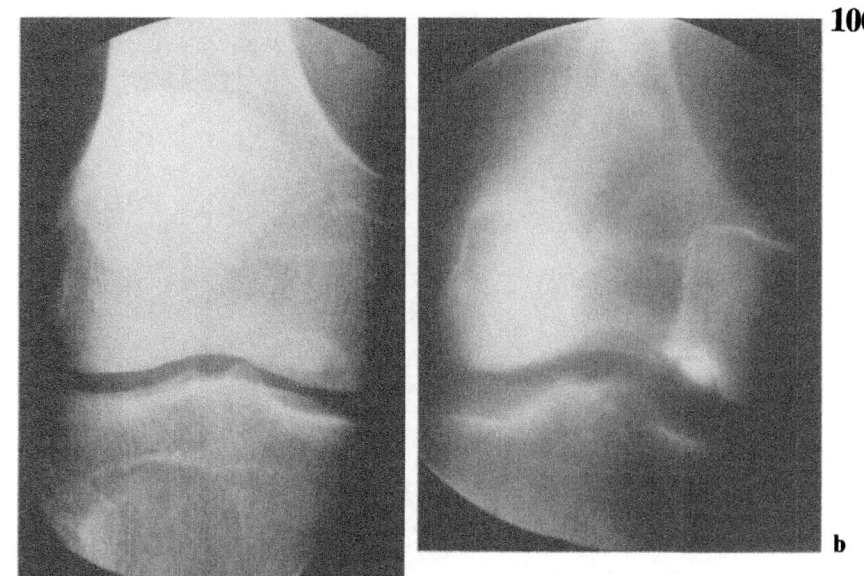

a

b

101

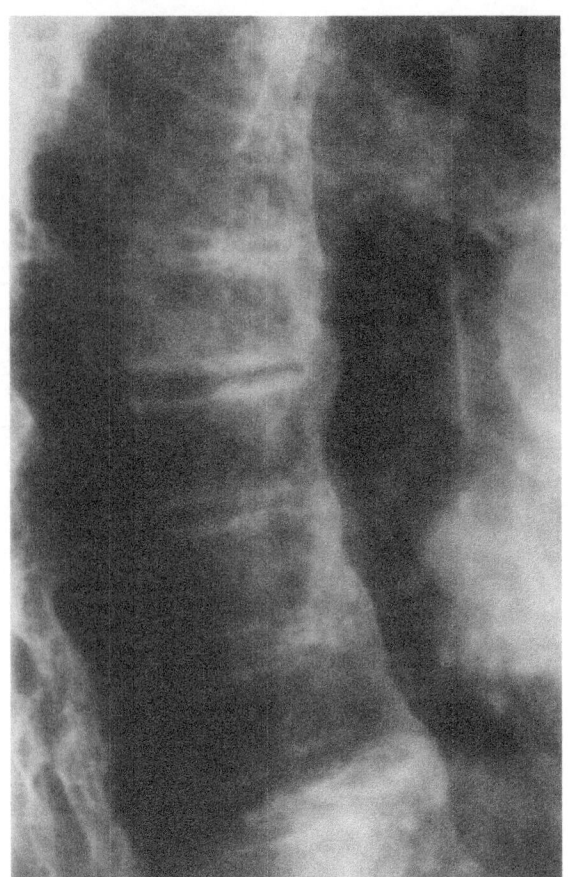

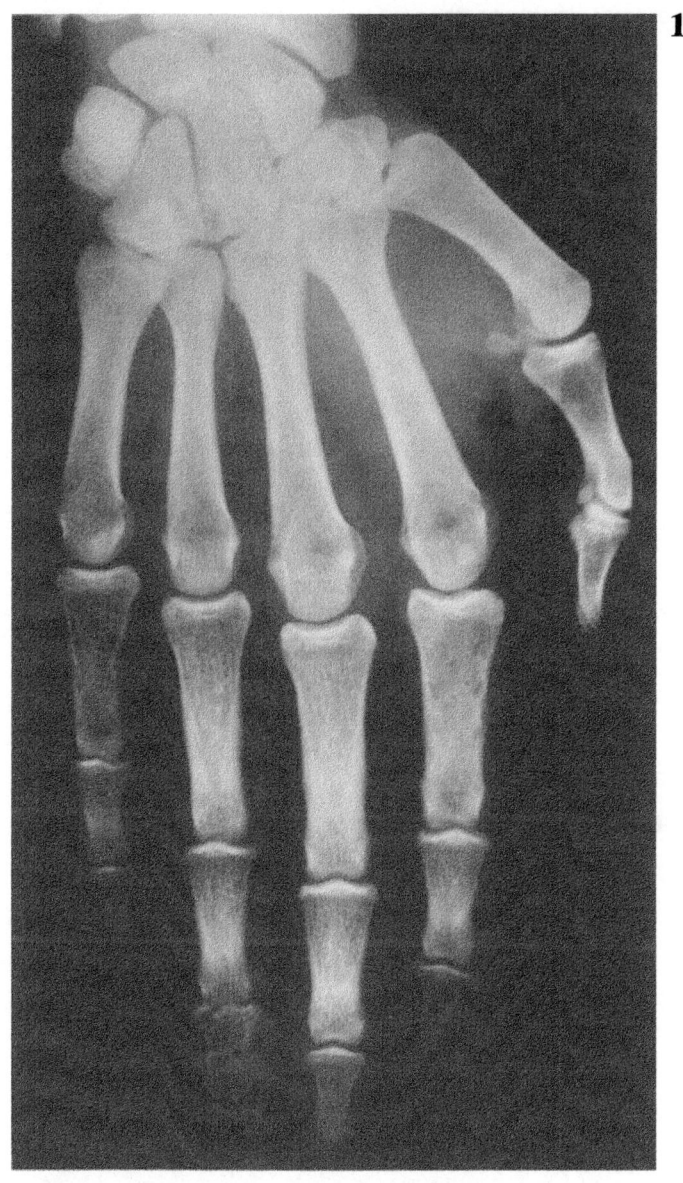

103

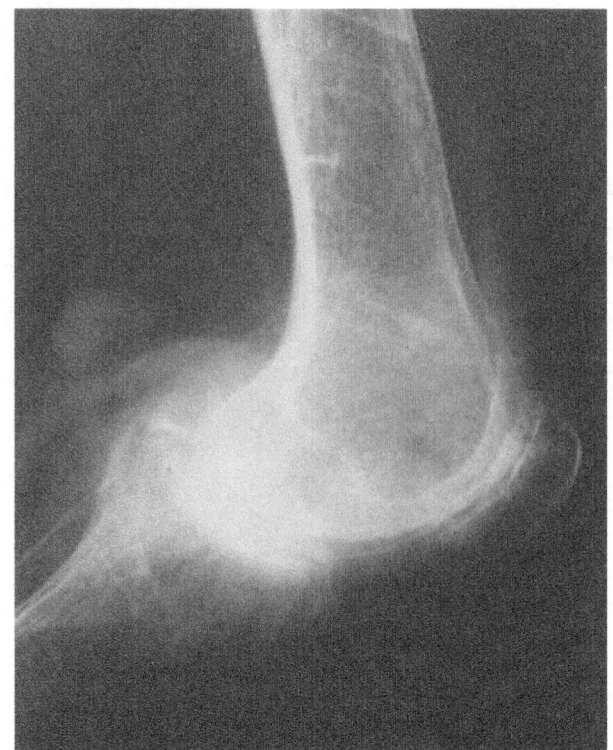

104

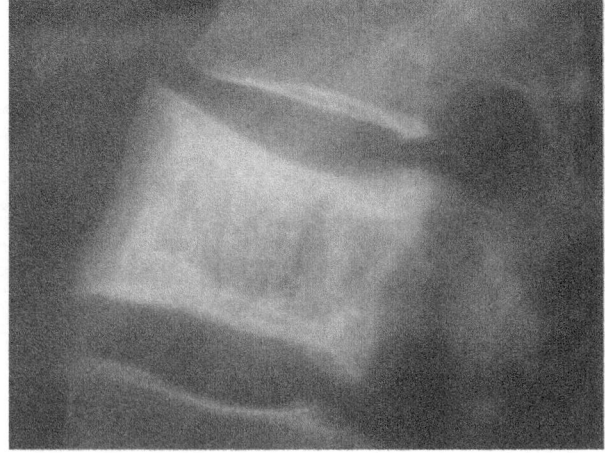

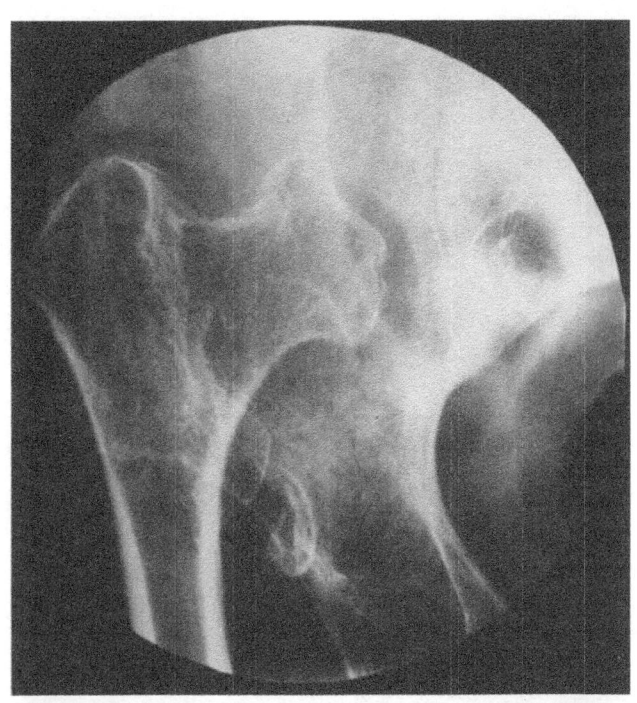

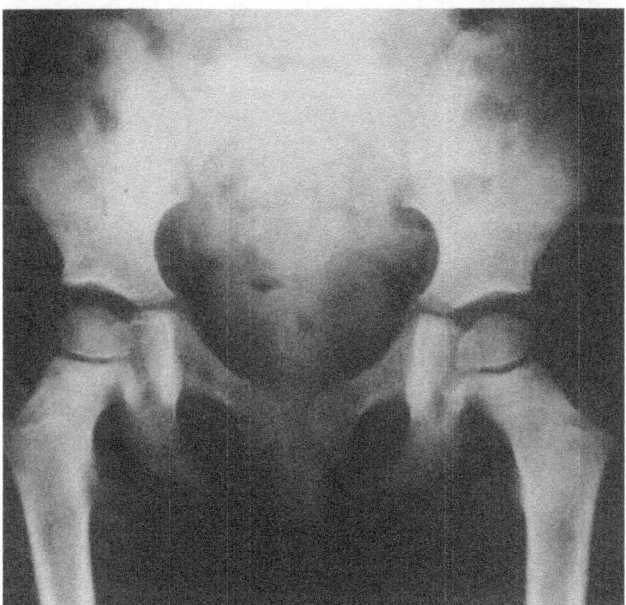

107-109

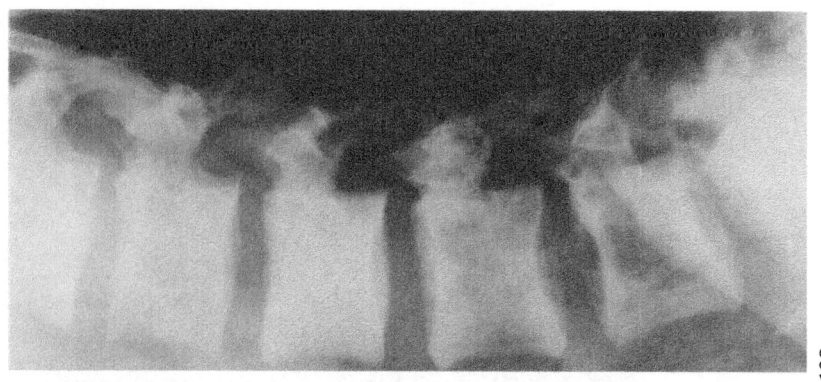

109

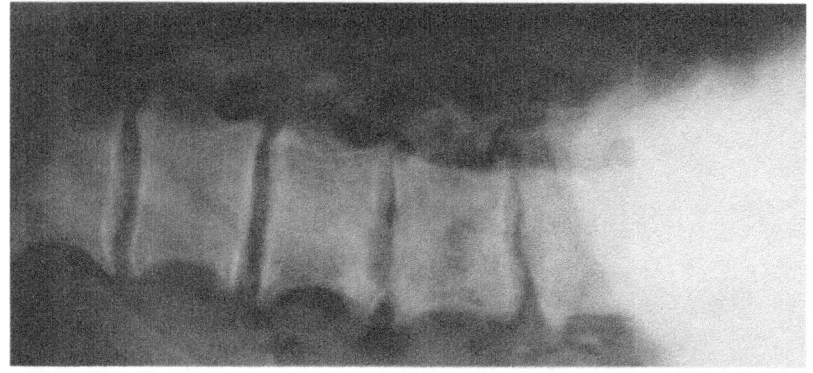

108

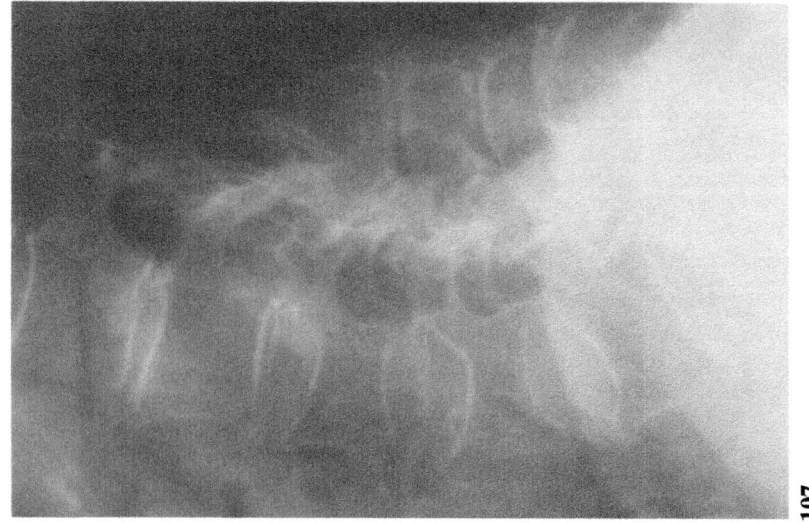

107

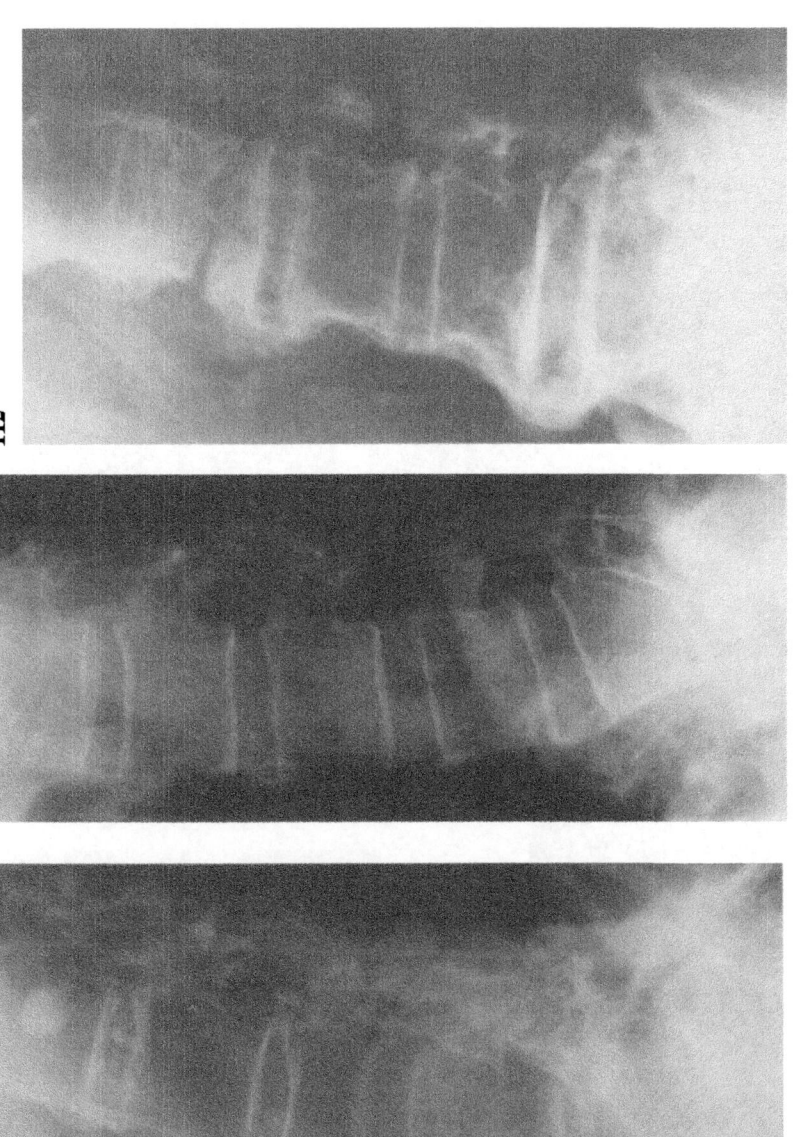

112

111

110

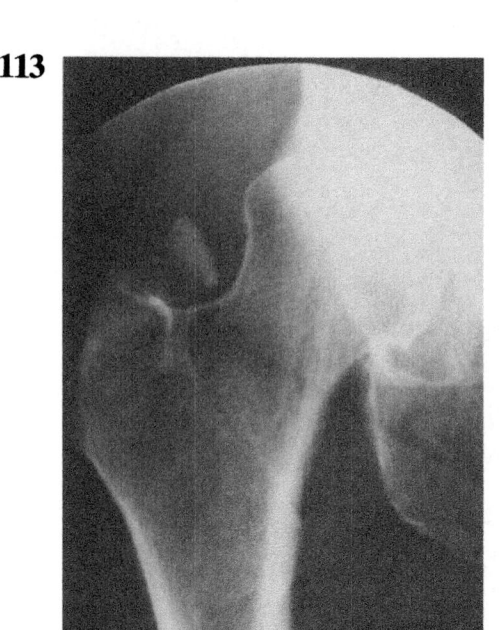

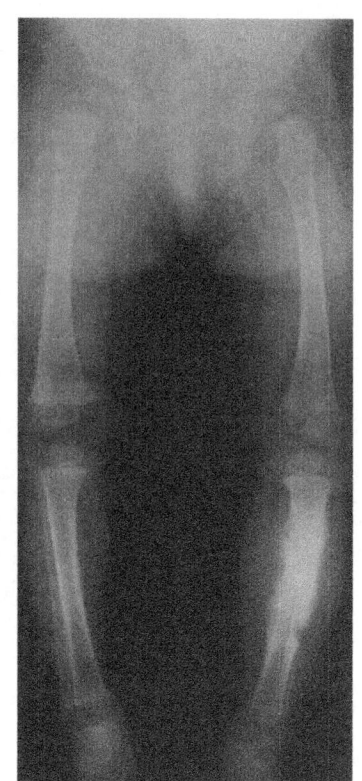

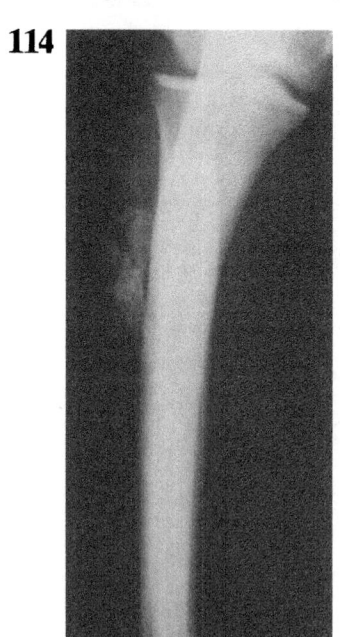

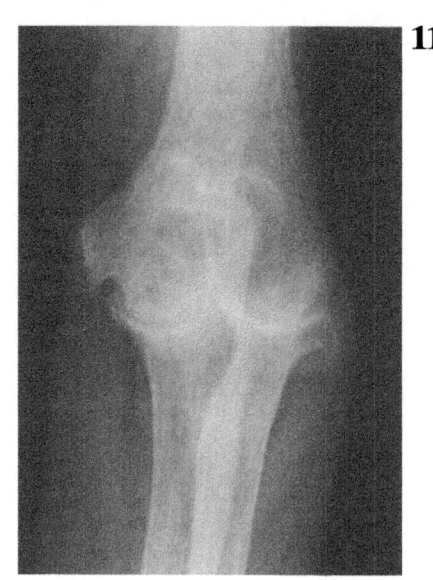

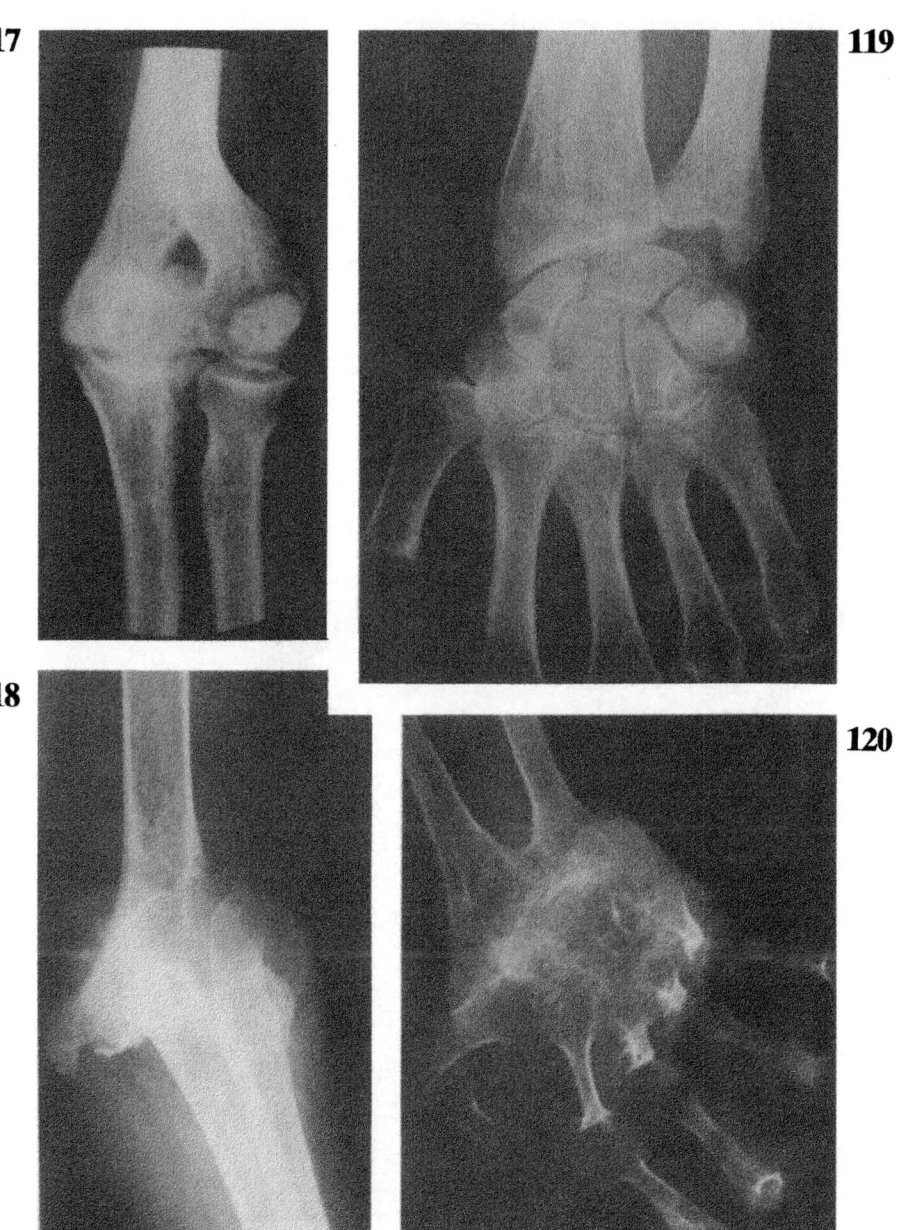

17

119

18

120

121

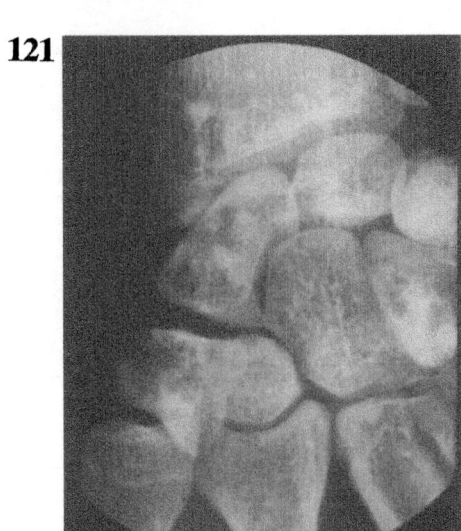

122

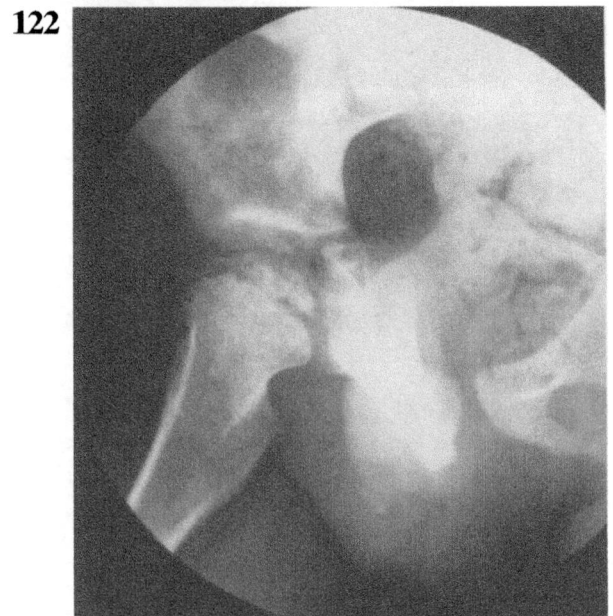

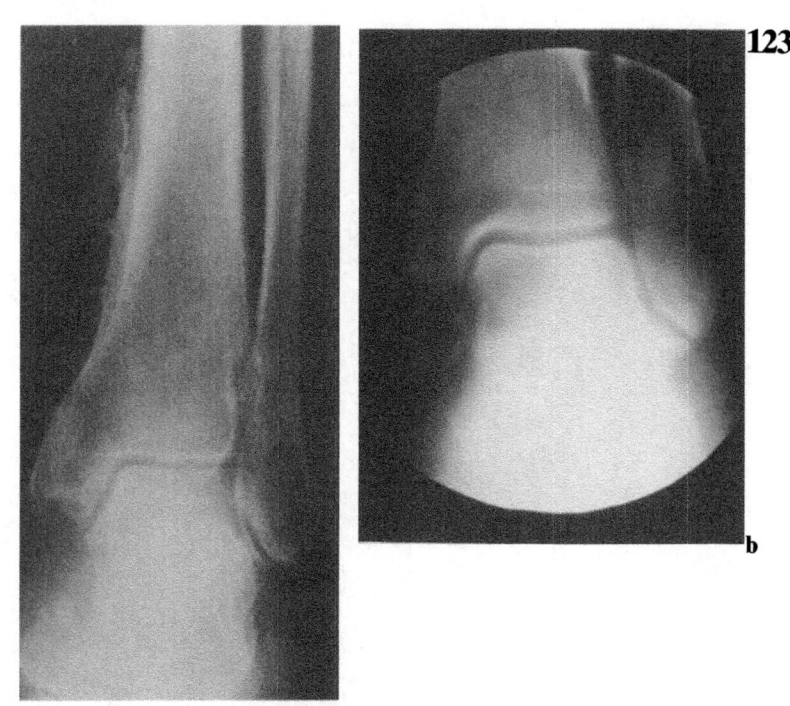

126

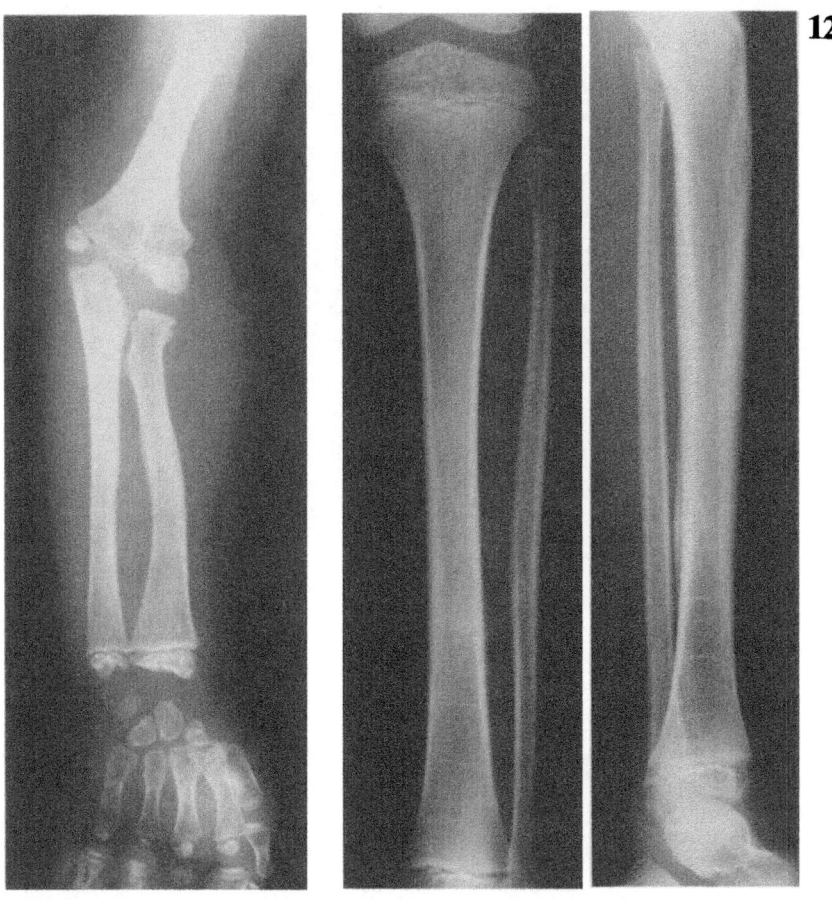

a   b

127

128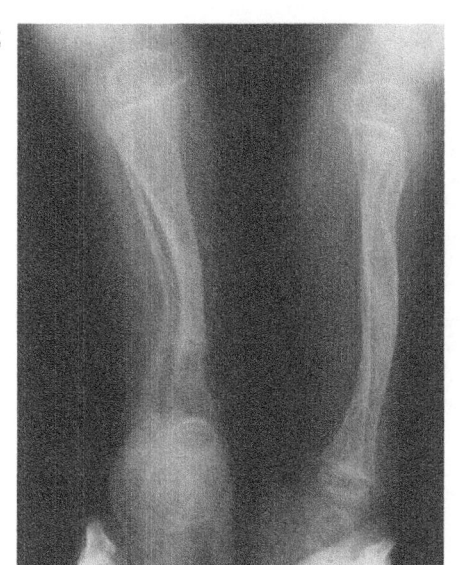

129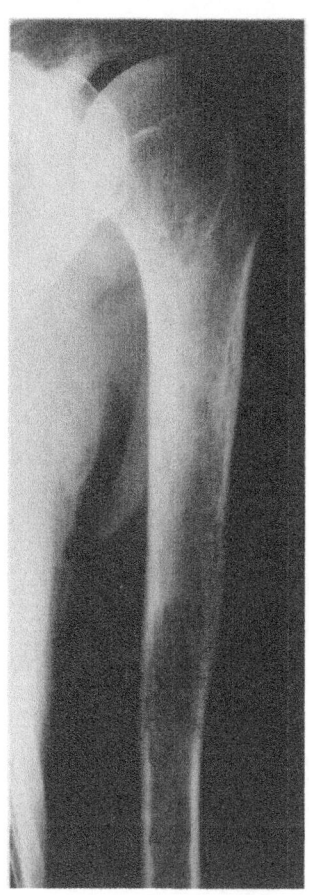

130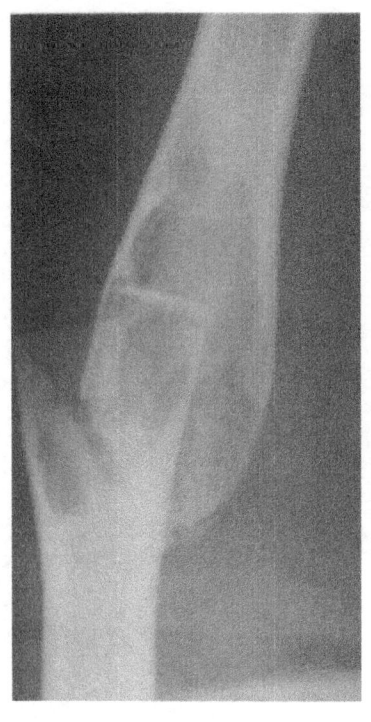

131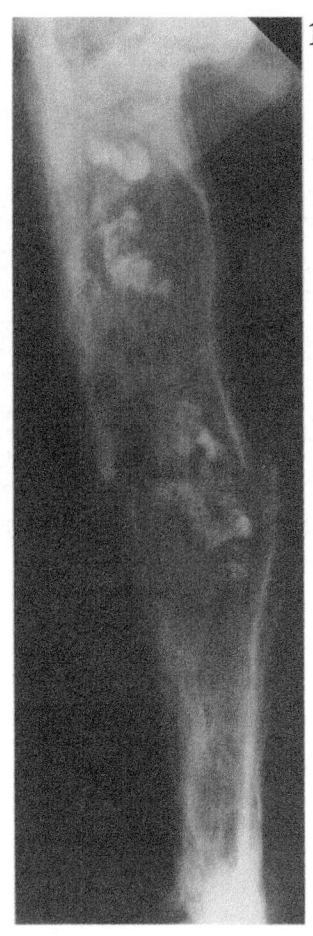

132

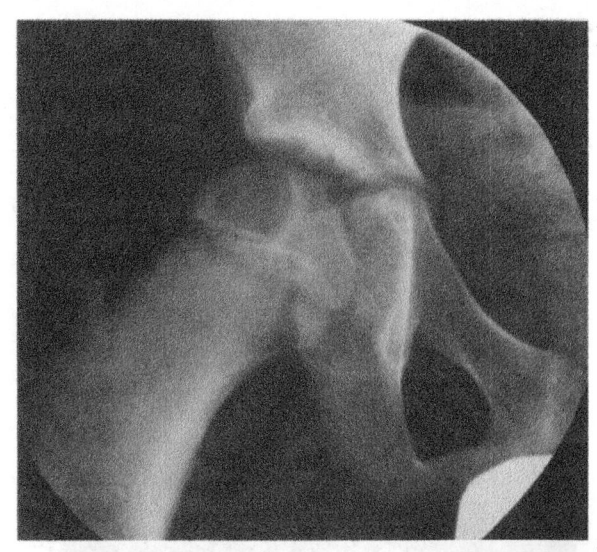

a

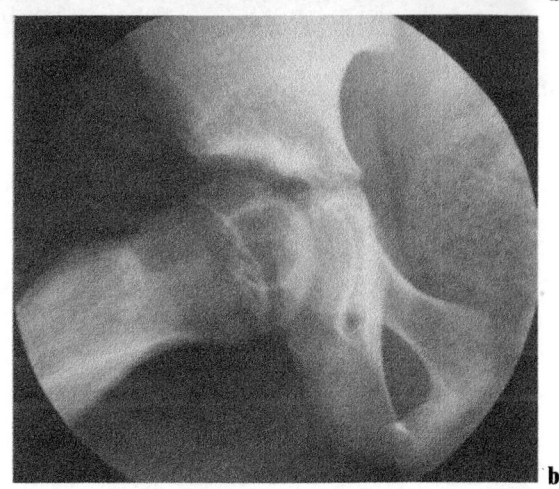

b

133

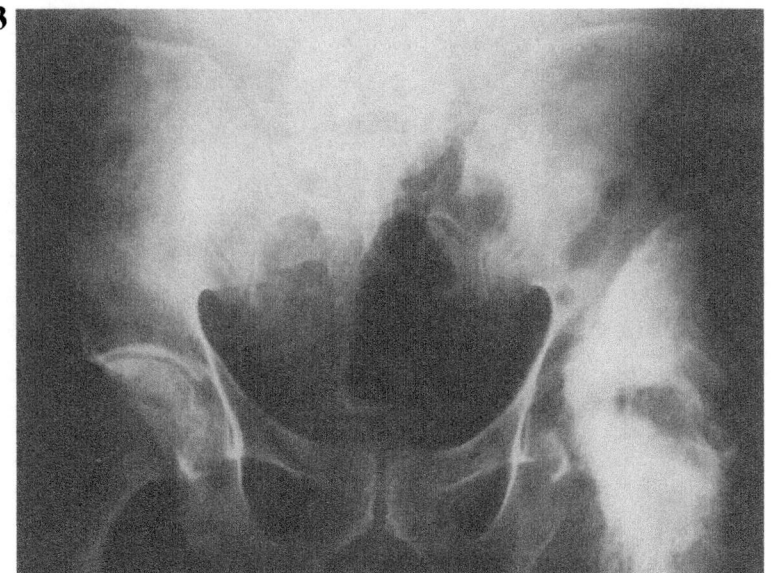

134

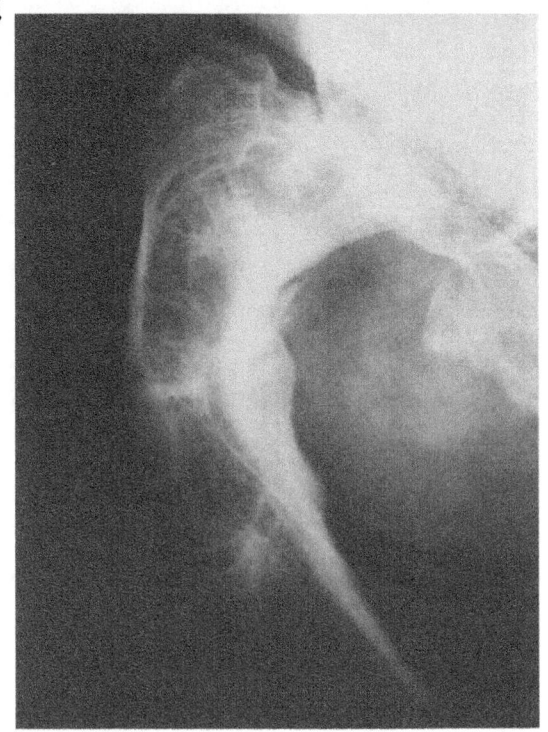

135

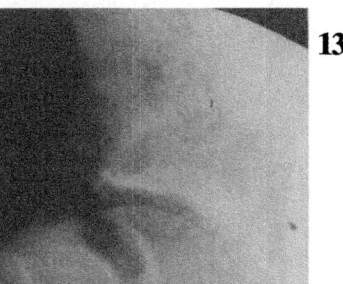

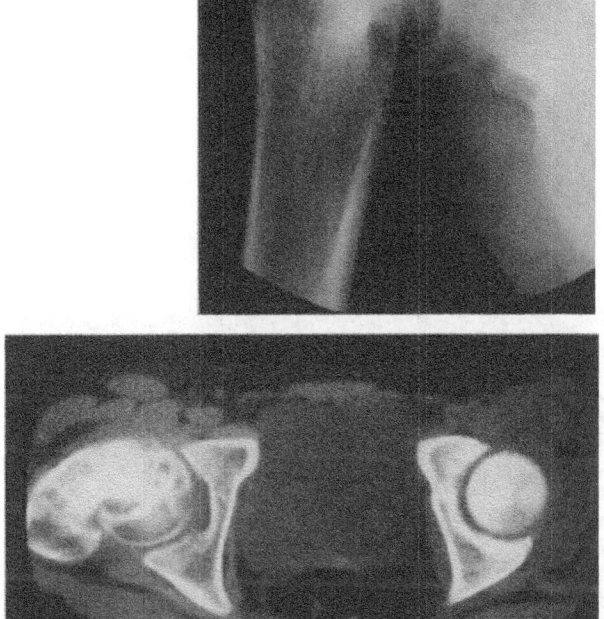

a

b

136
137

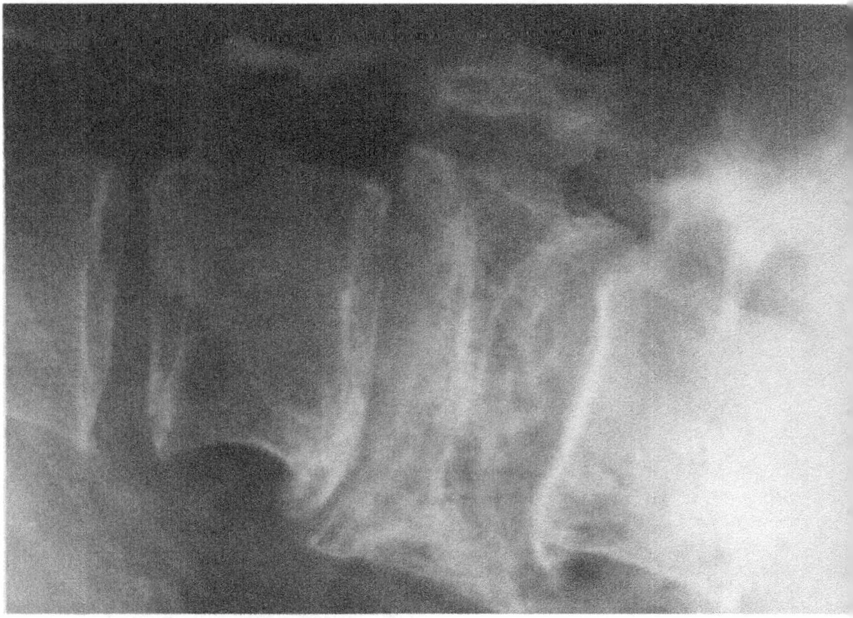

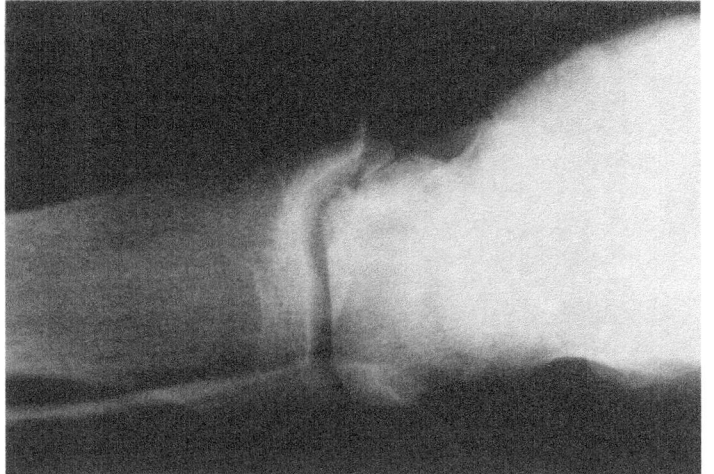

137

136

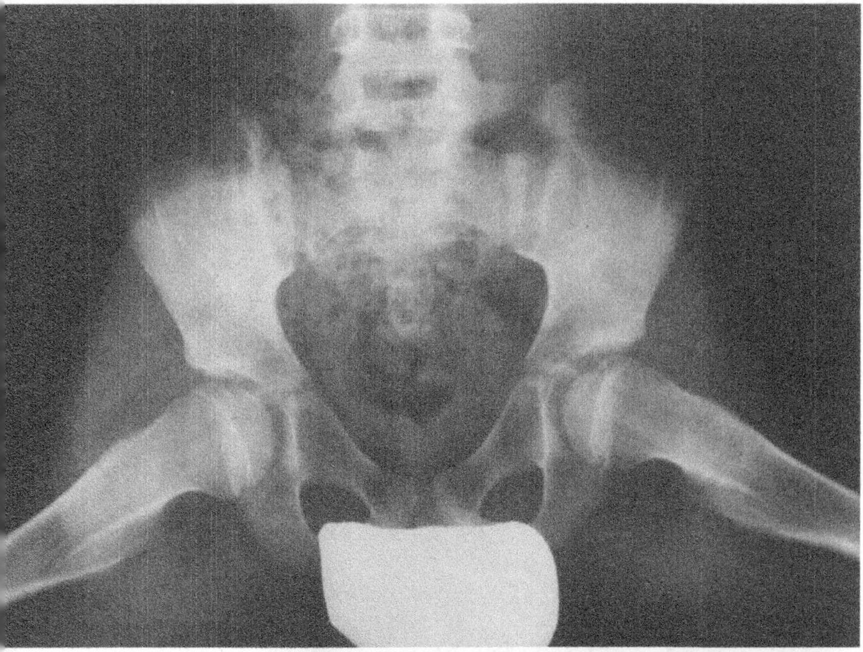

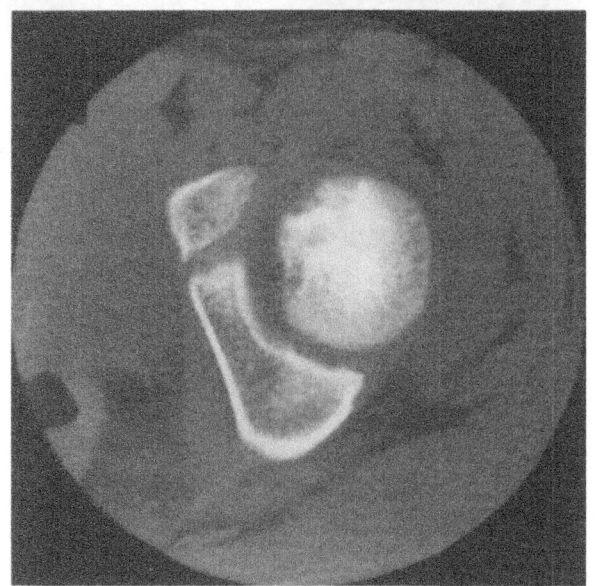

a

b

139

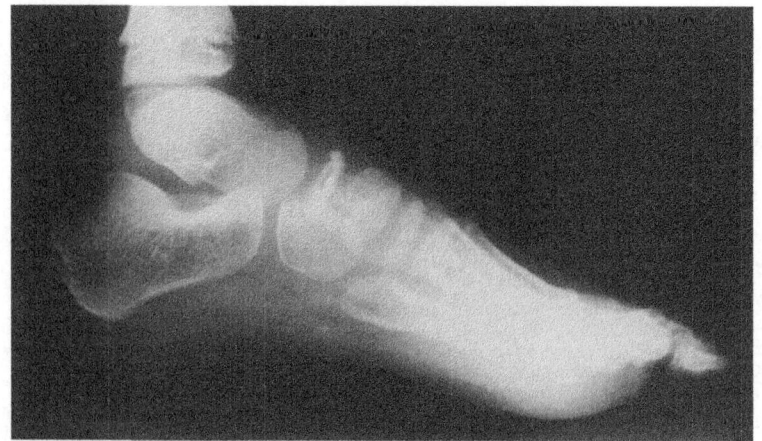

140

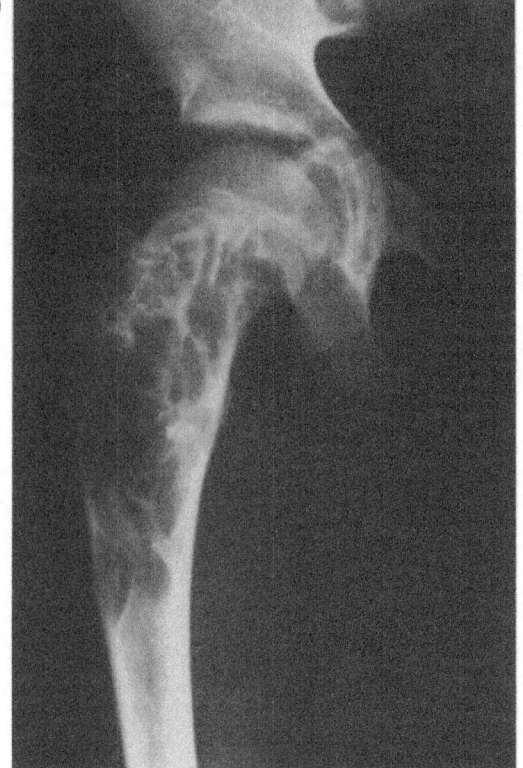

141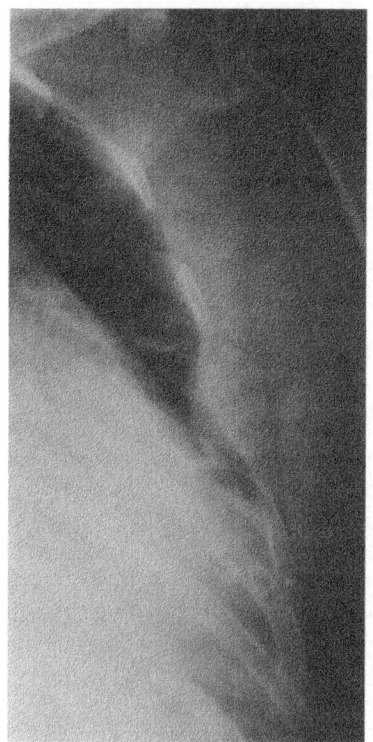

142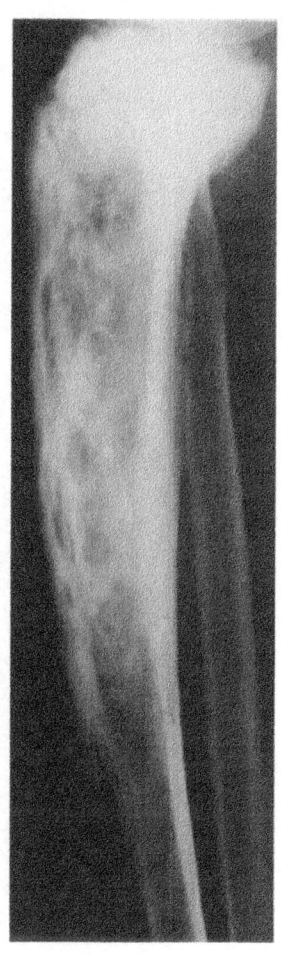

143

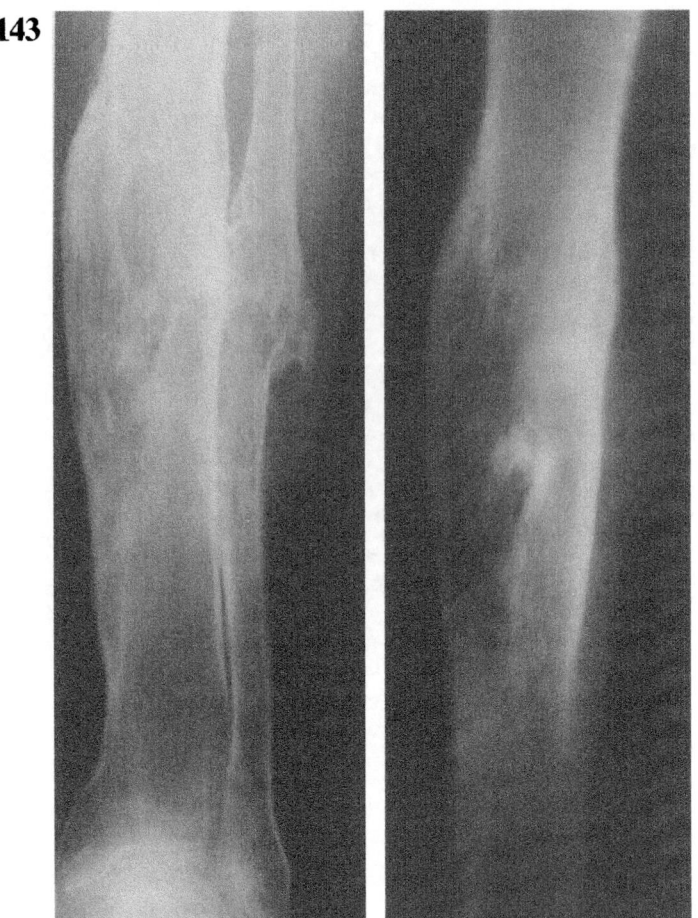

a   b

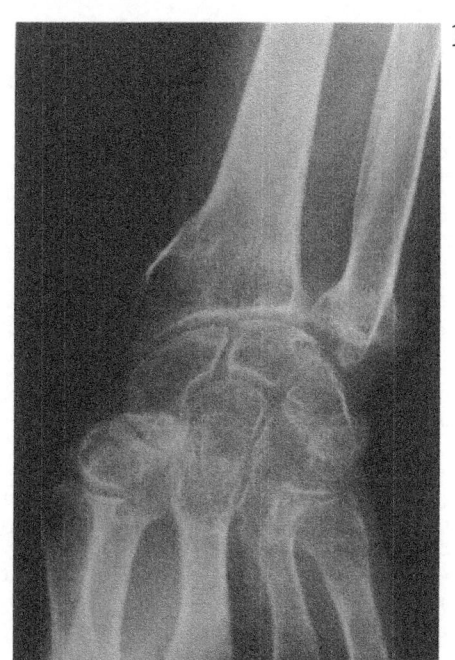

144

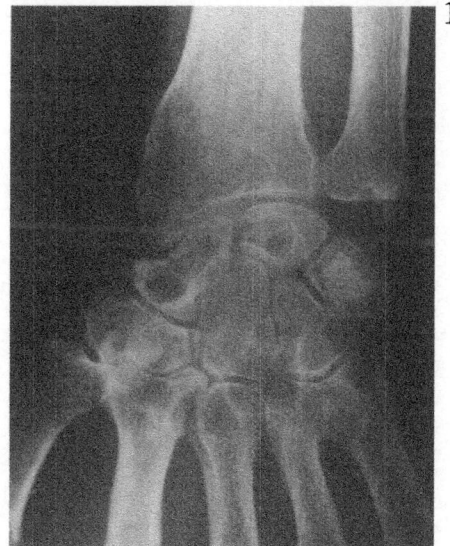

145

146

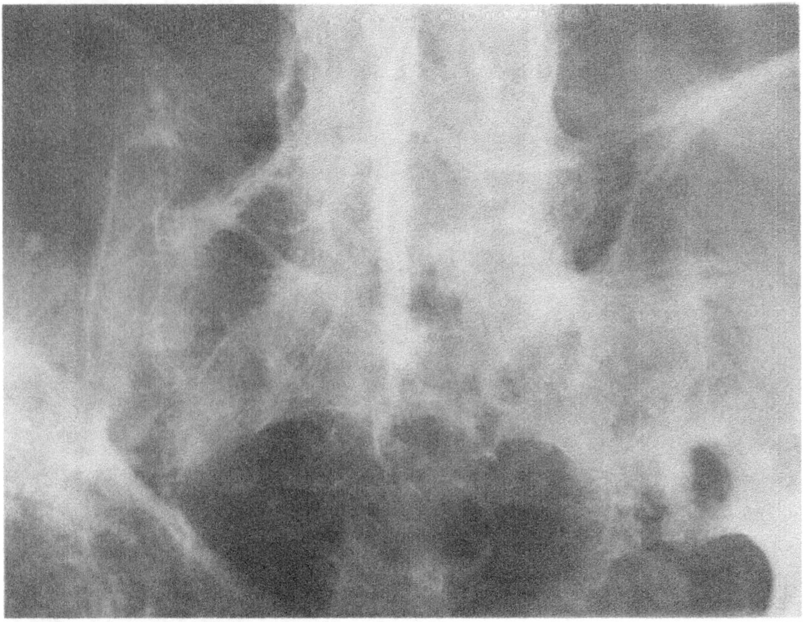

147

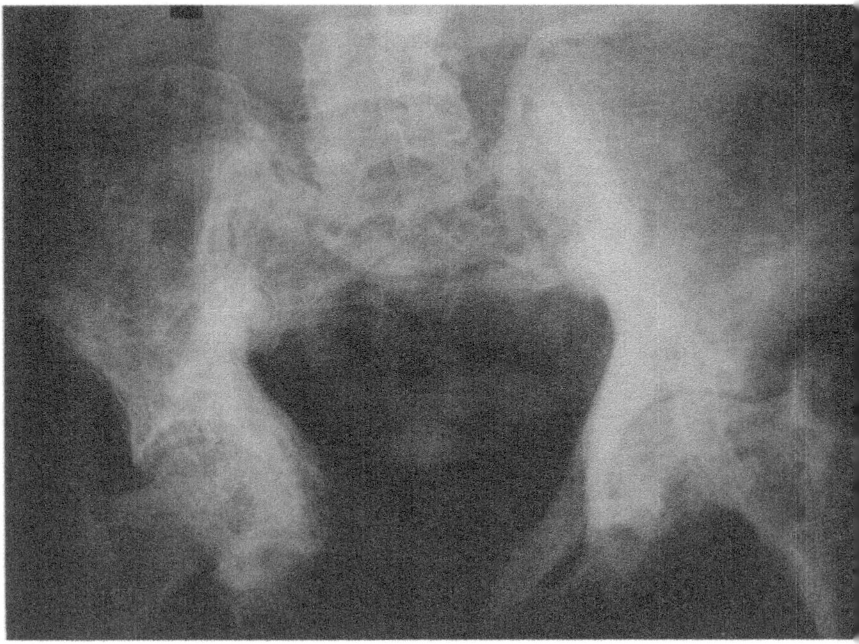

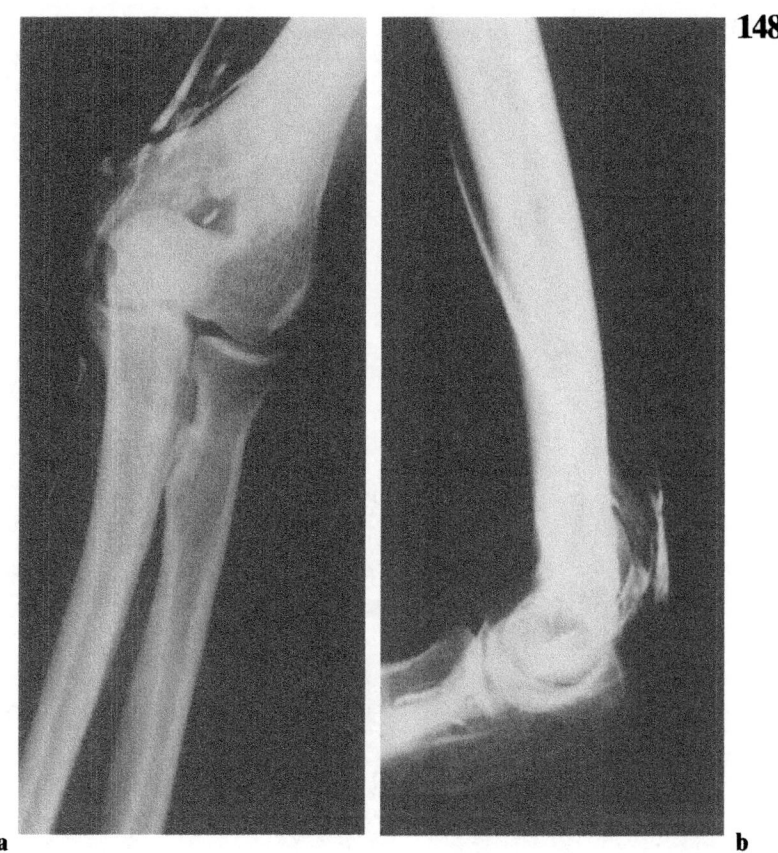

a   b

149

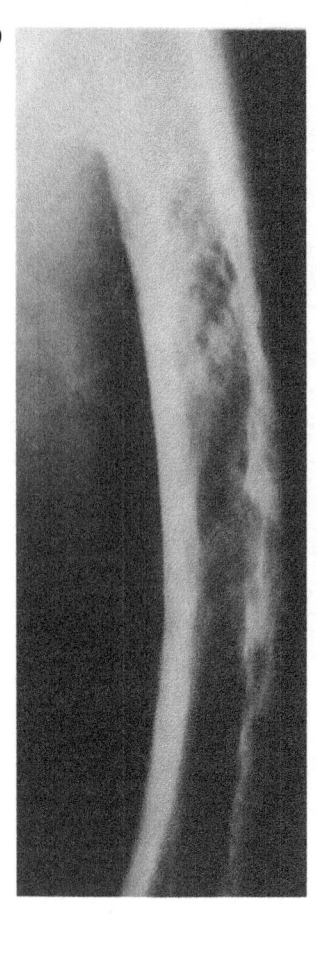

150

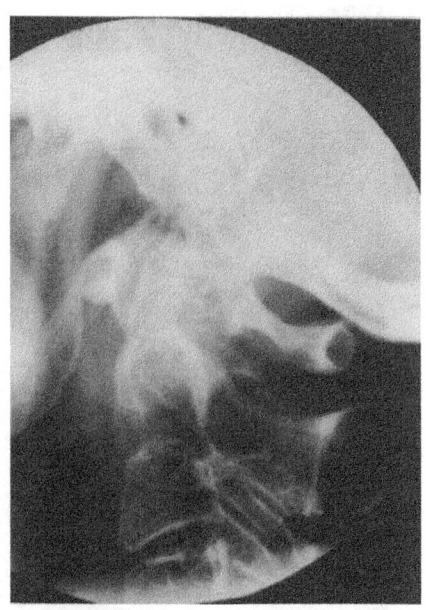

151

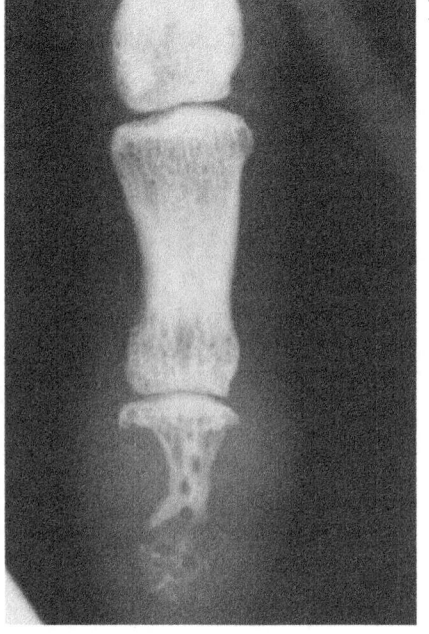

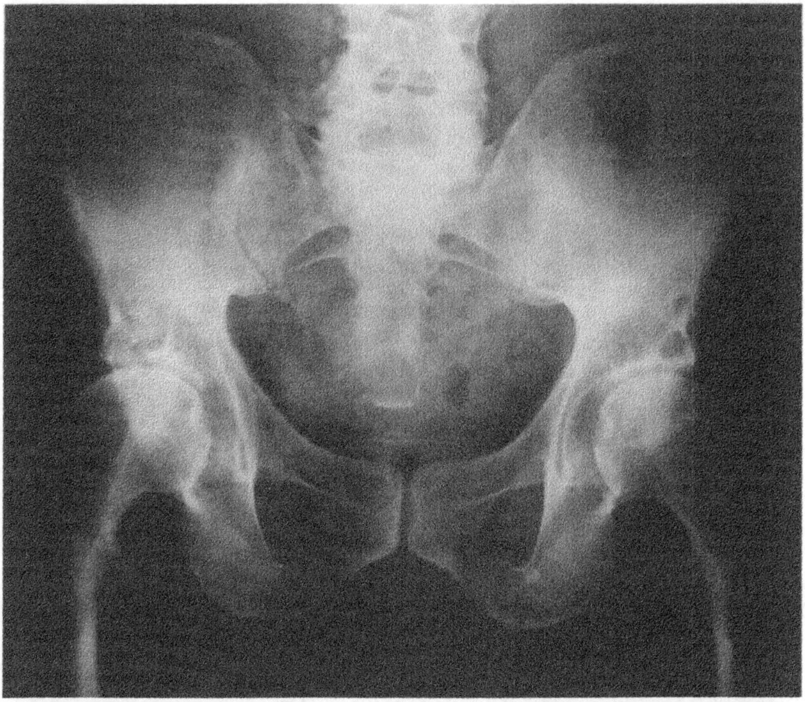

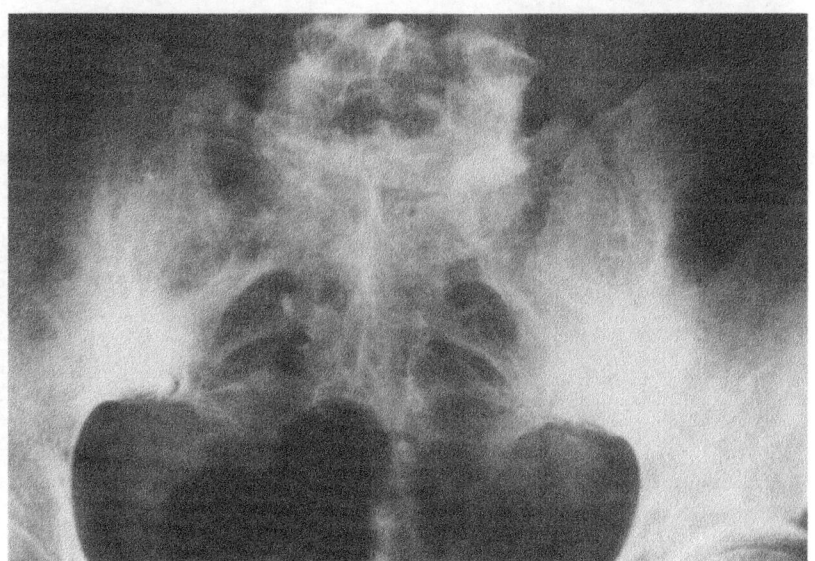

154

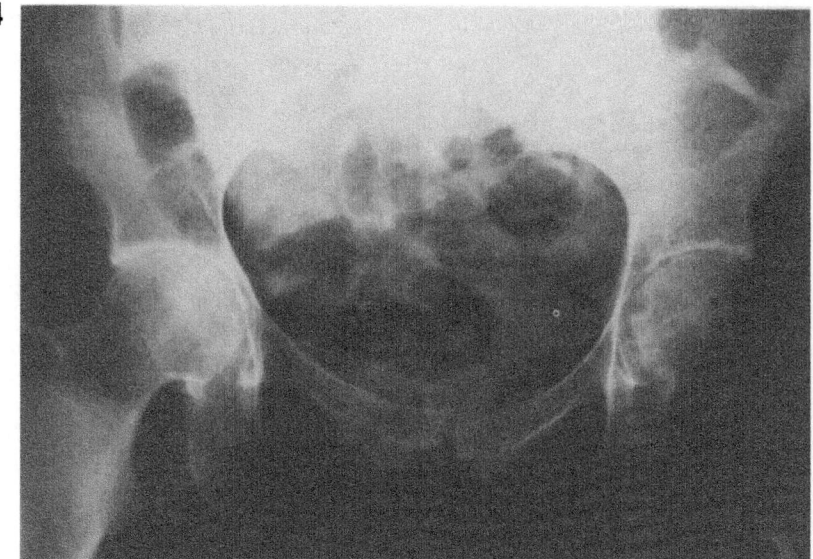

155

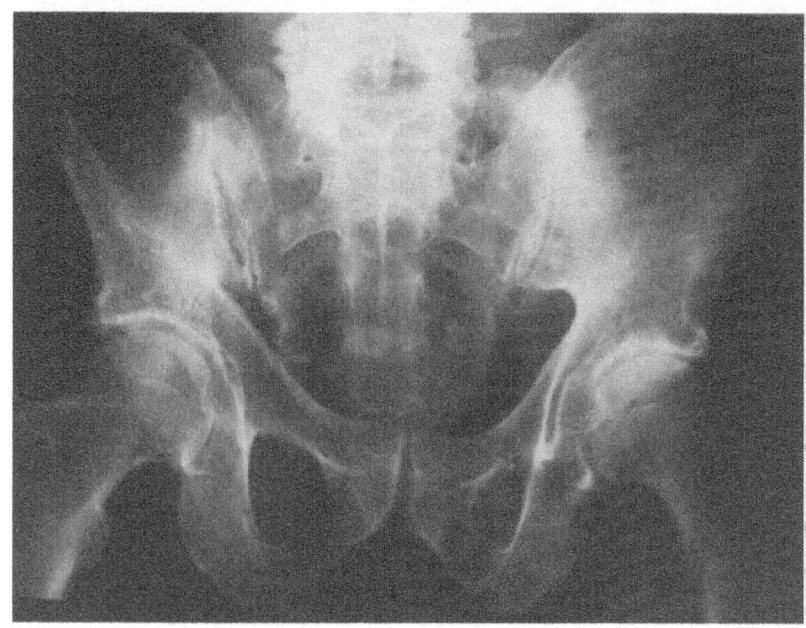

156

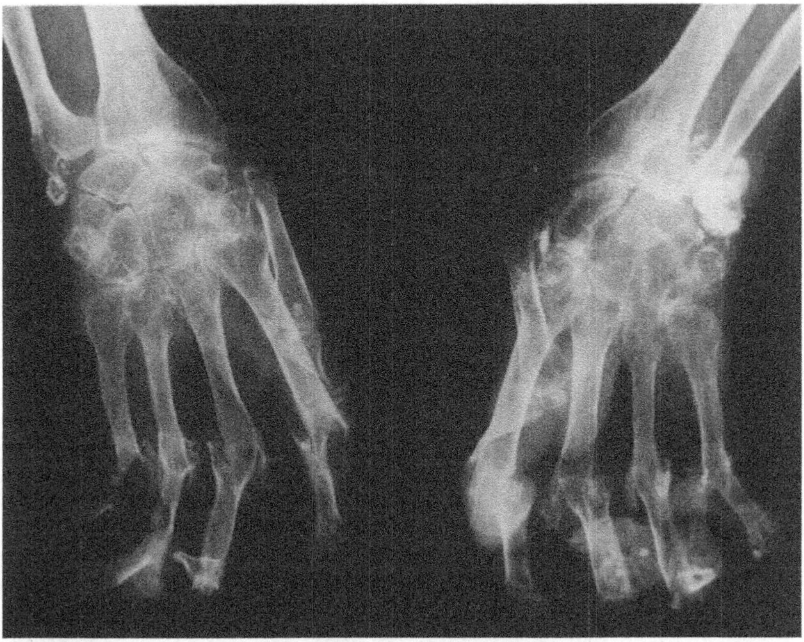

57

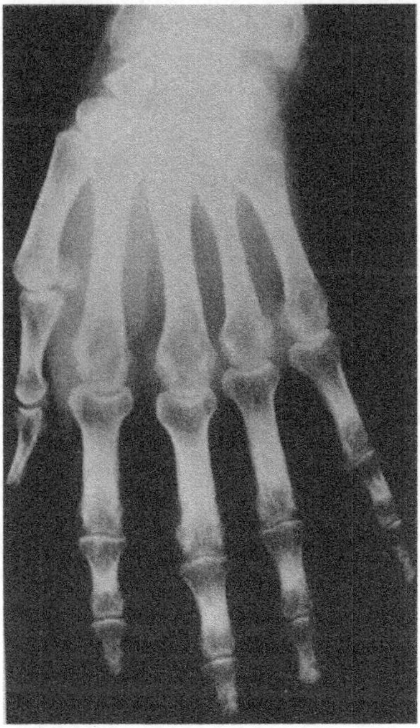

158

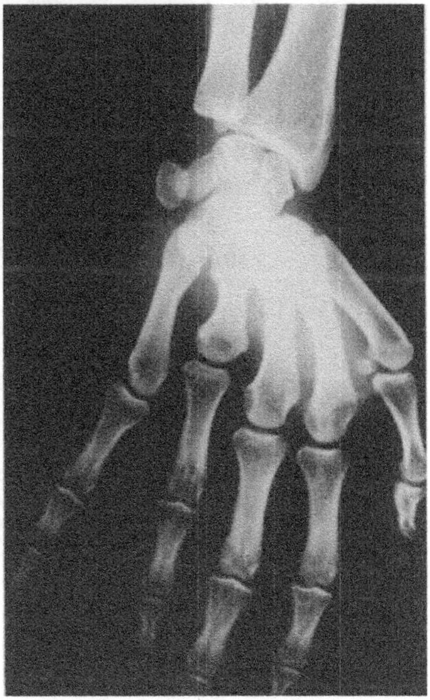

159
160

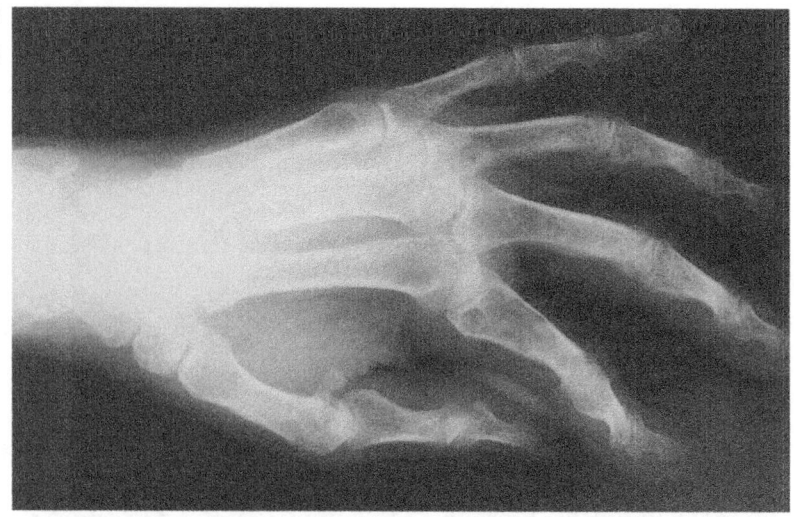

160

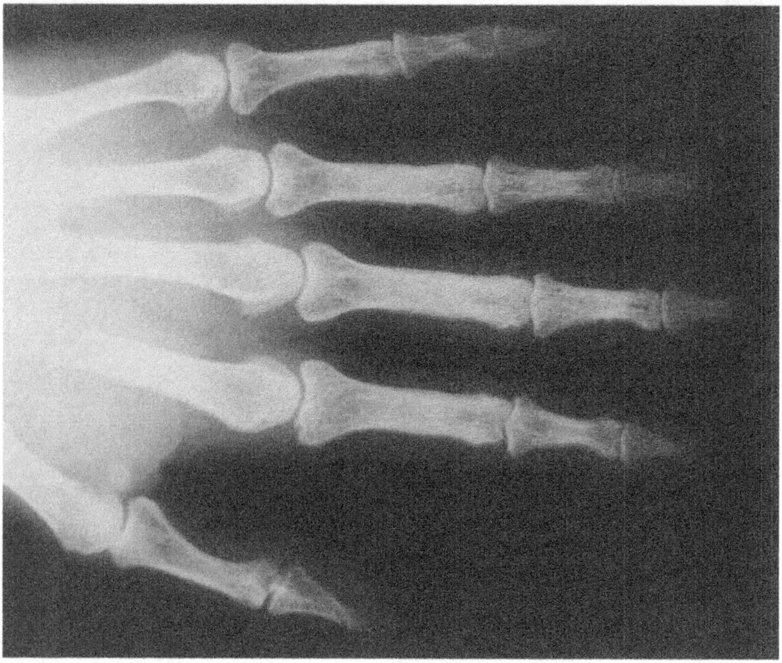

159

92

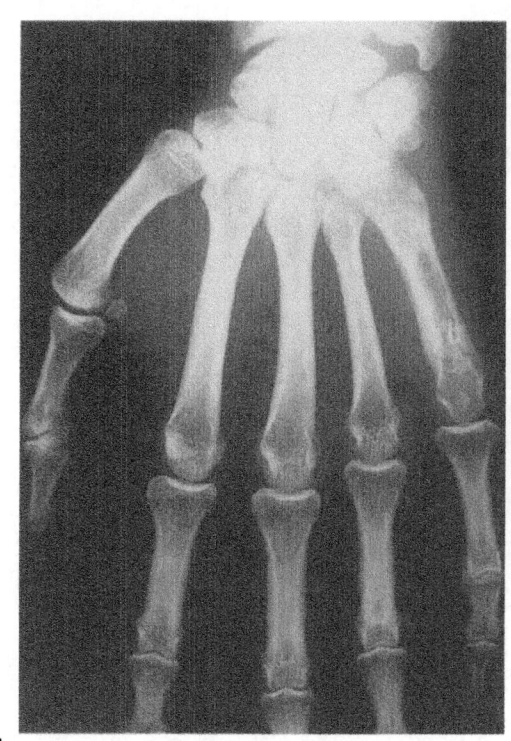

a

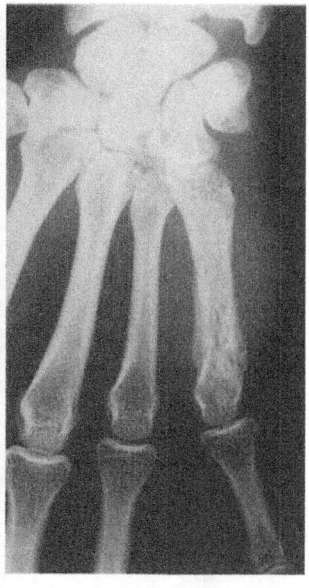

b

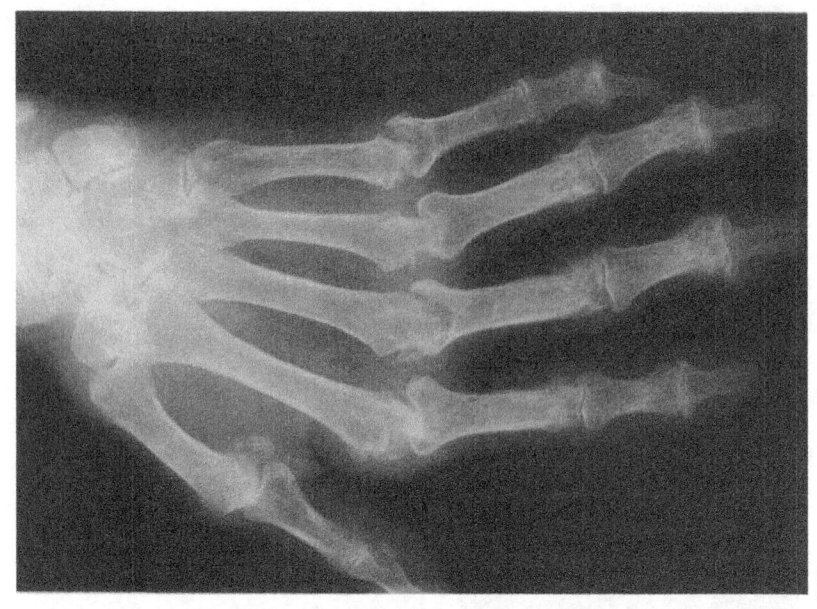

163

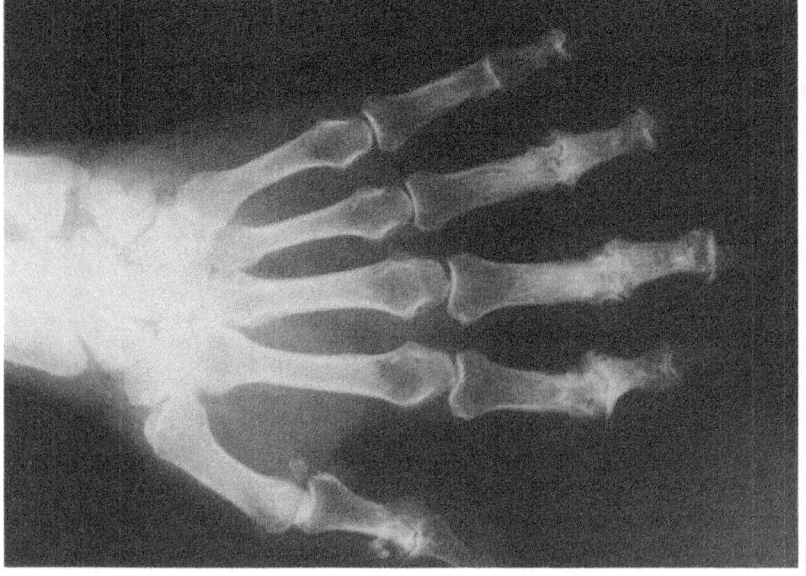

162

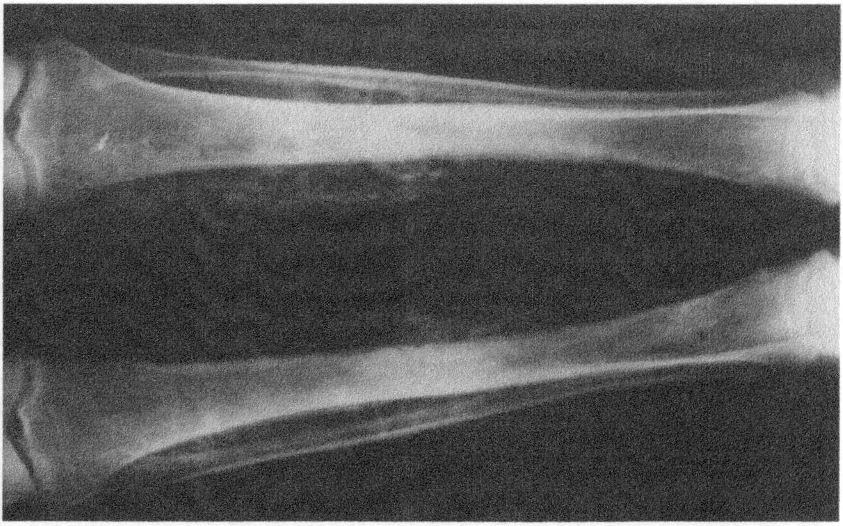

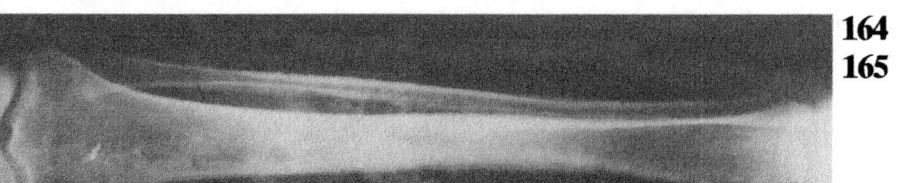

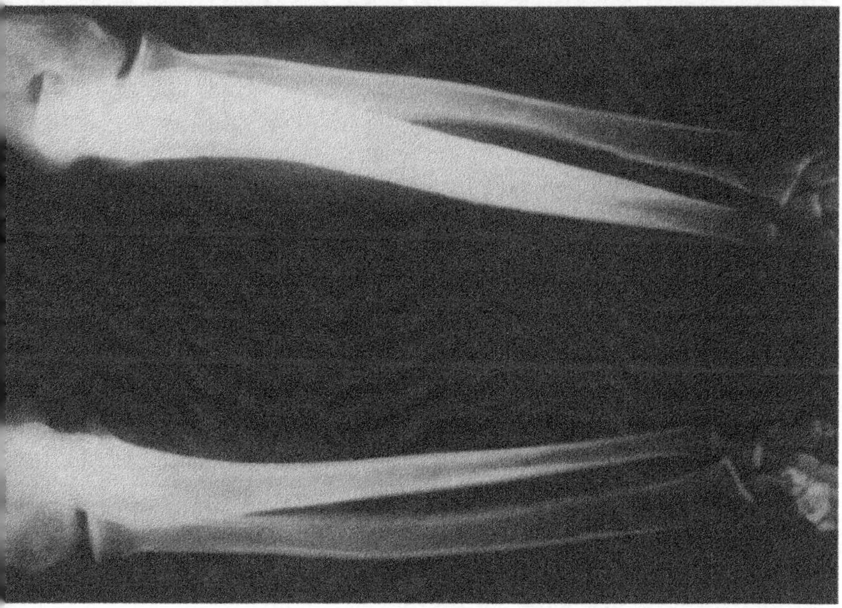

166

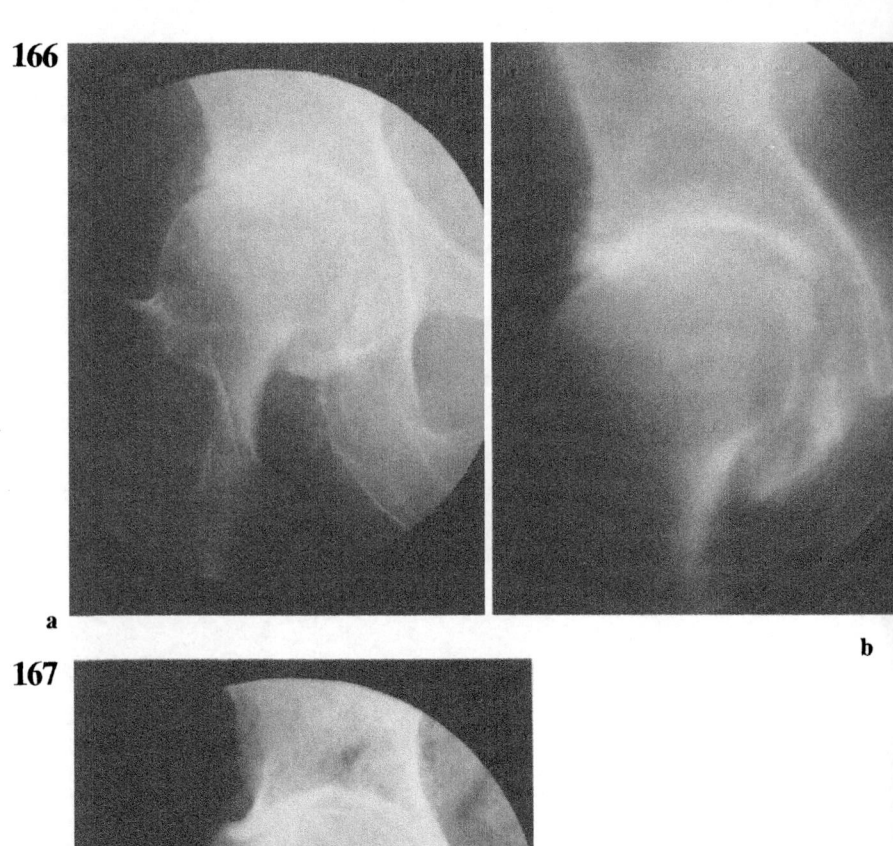

a

b

167

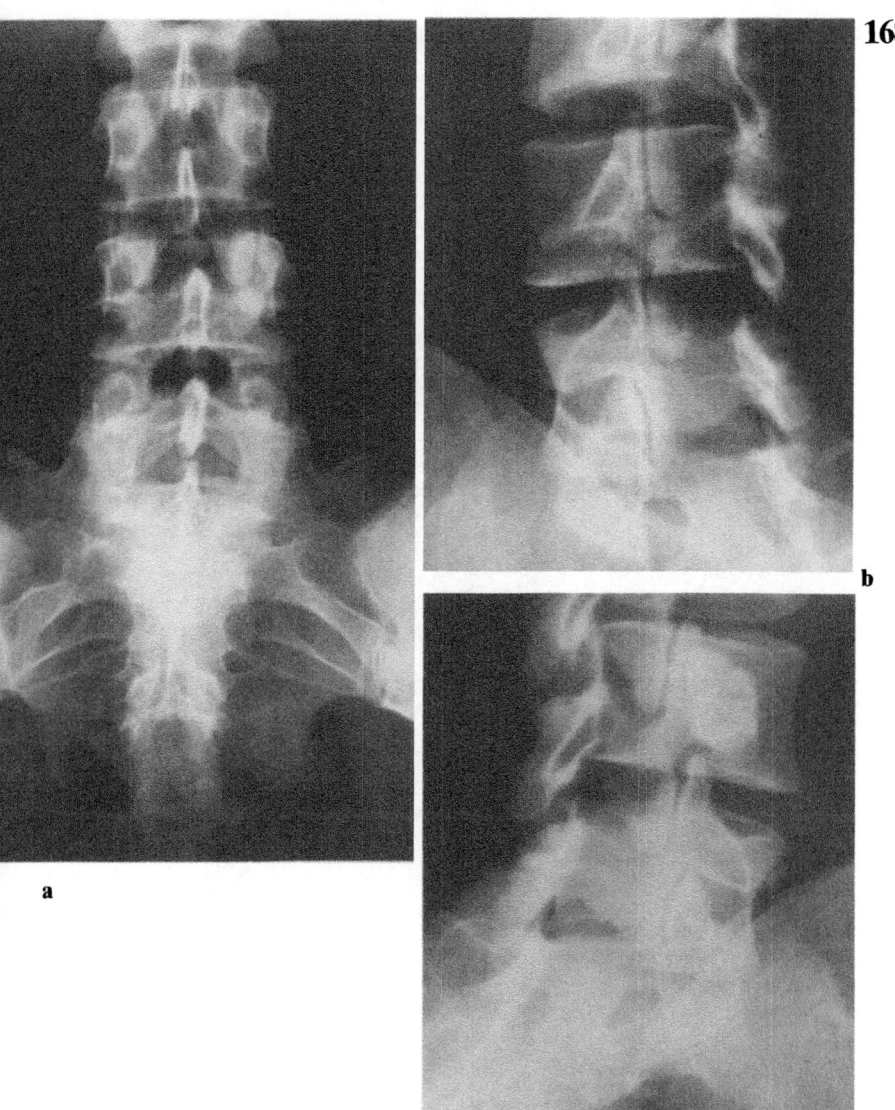

a

b

c

169

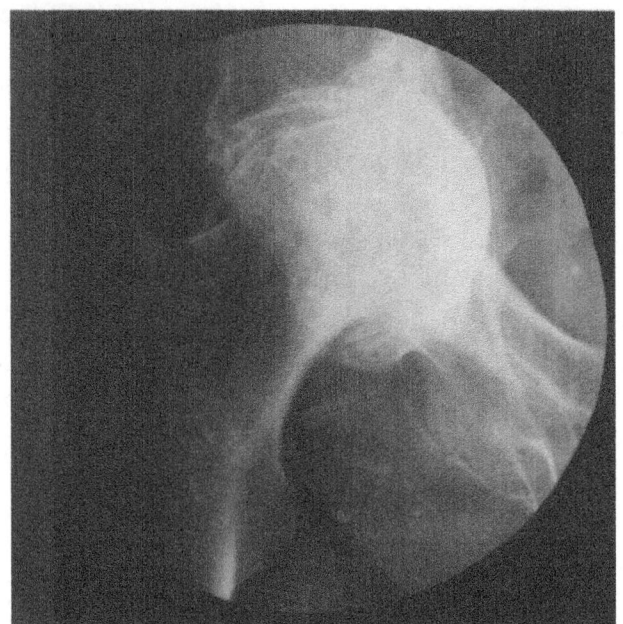

170

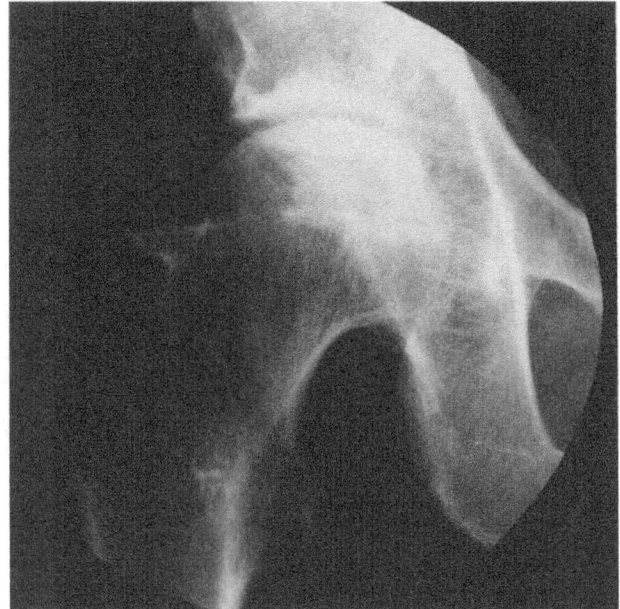

a

170

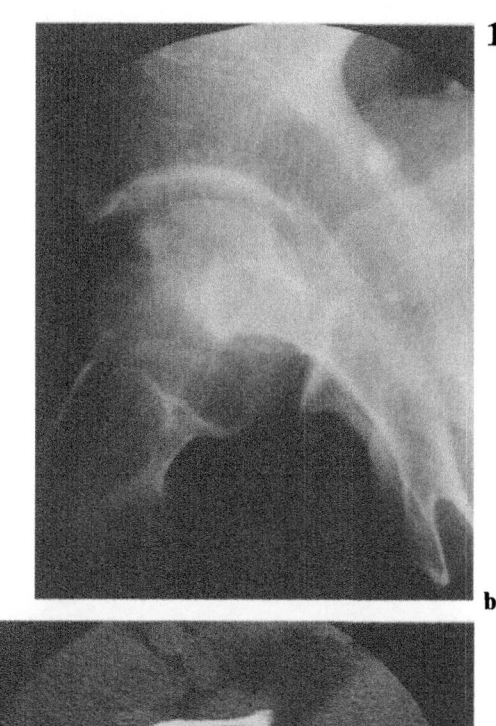

b

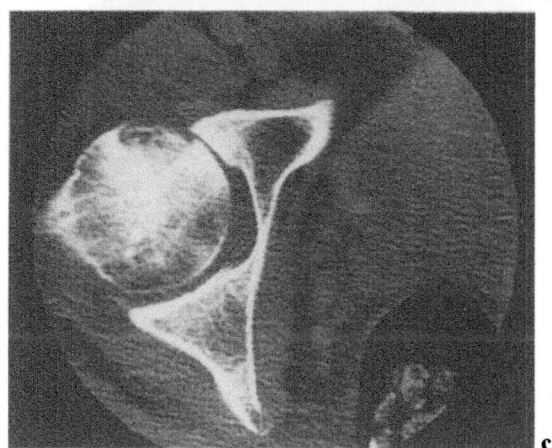

c

Part Two
Commentary with Corresponding Schemata

There is a well-defined lucent area with calcification in the proximal phalanx of the first toe. The cortex is moderately expanded. This appearance is pathognomic of *enchondroma* of the central type. This benign cartilaginous tumor occurs frequently. The phalanxes of the hand and feet are the most common sites. Multiple enchondromas occur in Ollier's disease (enchondromatosis) and in Mafucci's syndrome.

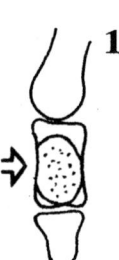

A chondroma is easily identified. It shows a double rupture of the cortex. There is a fracture through a central *chondroma*.

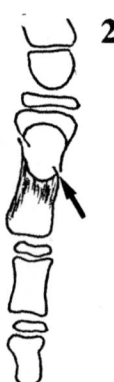

Enchondroma of the second phalanx, responsible for marked deformation of the cortex.

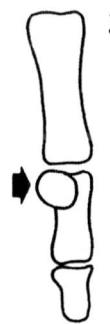

Fracture through a *chondroma*. These benign tumors are often detected incidentally following a fracture.

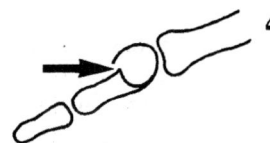

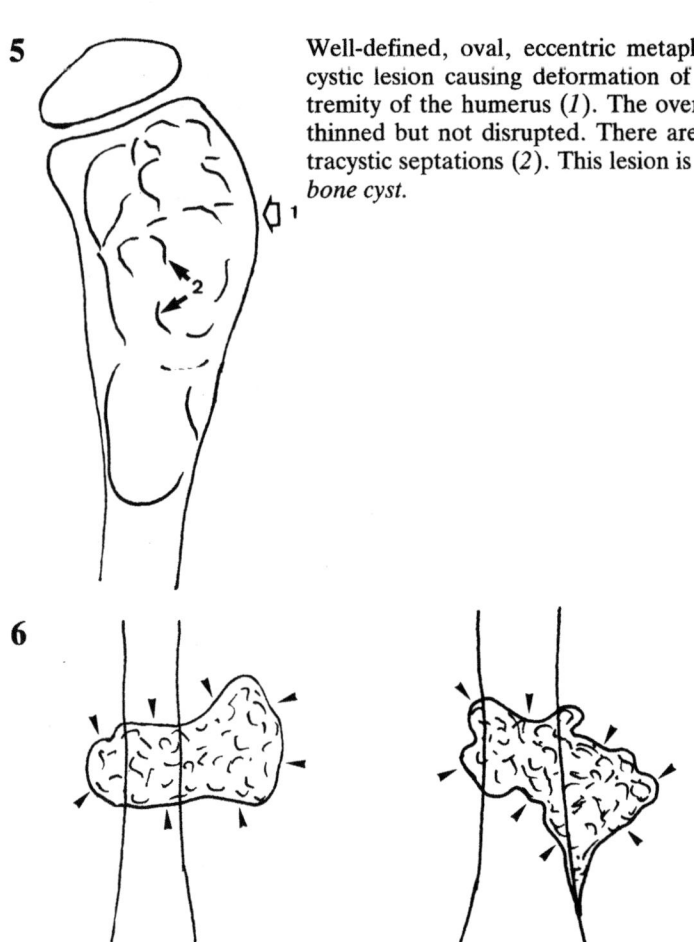

5 Well-defined, oval, eccentric metaphysodiaphyseal cystic lesion causing deformation of the upper extremity of the humerus (*1*). The overlying cortex is thinned but not disrupted. There are numerous intracystic septations (*2*). This lesion is an *aneurysmal bone cyst.*

6

Diaphyseal exostosis delimited by a well-defined cortex continuous with the cortex of the femoral diaphysis. The bone structure is alveolar with multiple septations. The adjacent soft tissues are displaced: There is no periosteal reaction. This lesion is an *osteochondroma* of the femoral diaphysis. The lesion is frequently larger than it appears to be on the radiogram. Often, a noncalcified tumor of considerable size lies beneath the calcification. In adults, this cartilaginous area tends to involute. It is potentially malignant, but this is a rare complication. Growth or soft tissue calcification beyond the lesion may indicate incipient malignant change.

Vertebral angioma. The body of L3 has an alveolar structure. The cortices are well-defined and the vertebral plates are unaffected. The posterior arch shows the same features. Note the defect of the posterior arch of L5; it has no pathological significance.

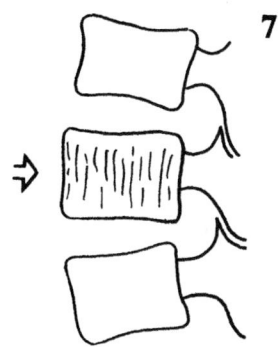

Bone infarct. Irregular and sinuous metaphysodiaphyseal opacity located in the medullary cavity. Bone infarcts are often asymptomatic and discovered incidentally. Bone necrosis results in devitalized bone, which may subsequently undergo calcification. Infarcts in bone are mainly located in the diaphyses of the bones of the lower limbs and may involve one or several bones.

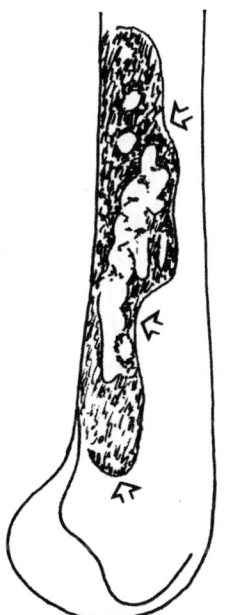

Osteoblastic disease of the spine.

Standard radiographs (**a**) show thoracolumbar scoliosis. They are otherwise normal. Radionuclide scanning (**b**) shows increased uptake of the tracer in the area of T11. CT scan (**c**), with an axial section through the plane of the vertebral body, shows a lucent area with a sclerotic margin at the level of the right lamina of T11. This appearance strongly suggests *osteoid osteoma.* Osteoid osteoma is a cause of painful scoliosis. The lesion is located on the apex of the concavity.

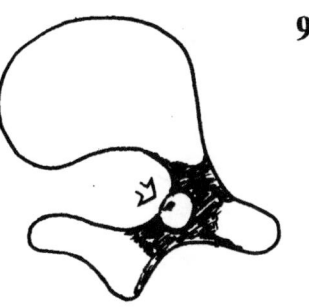

10

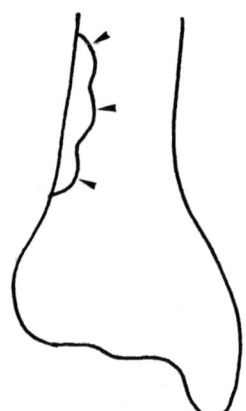

Metaphyseal, eccentric, oval radiolucent area with vertical long axis. Its endosteal margin is well-defined and serpiginous with peripheral sclerosis. This appearance is pathognomonic of *cortical defect*.

11

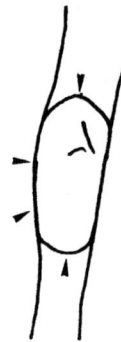

Eosinophilic granuloma.

– Radiolucent central oval area is shown with clearly defined limits;
– the cortex is eroded from inside outwards and thinned;
– the diaphysis is expanded.

These features define eosinophil granuloma of the long bones.

12

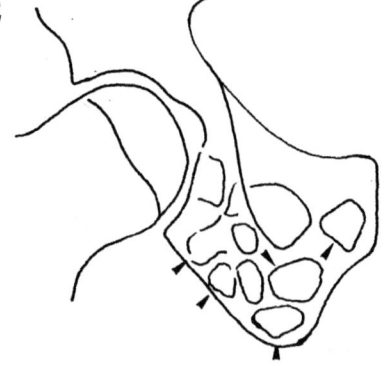

Myeloma located on the ischiopubic ramus. Juxtaposition of well-circumscribed rounded and oval lesions without surrounding sclerosis. There are no signs of bone structure within the lesions.

Osteogenic fibroma, or benign osteoblastoma.

13

Well-circumscribed lucent area with expanded cortex (*1*) and surrounding sclerosis (*2*). There is some intralesional ossification, a sign that the lesion is longstanding (*3*). This tumor involves the spine first, and then the long bones of the limbs.

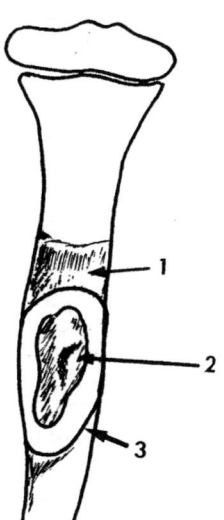

Aneurysmal bone cyst.

14

Expanding osteolytic lesion located in the metaphysis. The cortex is deformed and thinned, but not disrupted. The lucent area is finely trabeculated.

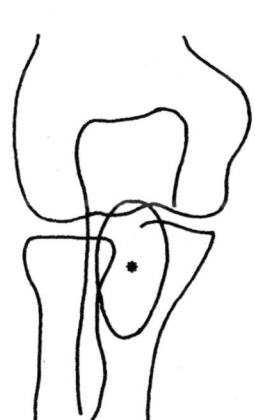

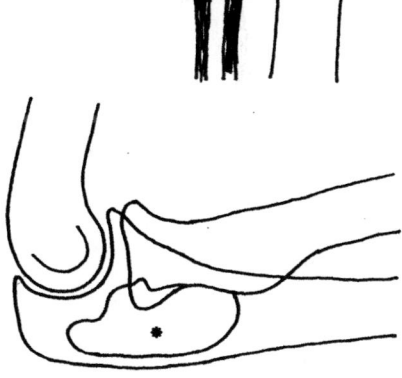

15

Villonodular synovitis of the elbow, or benign synovioma.

Homogeneous lucent area with well-defined margins, located in the epiphysometaphyseal region. The tumor does not deform, and the cortex is normal. This benign neoplasm is characterized by hyperplastic synovia with secondary epiphyseal bone lesions due to erosion.

16

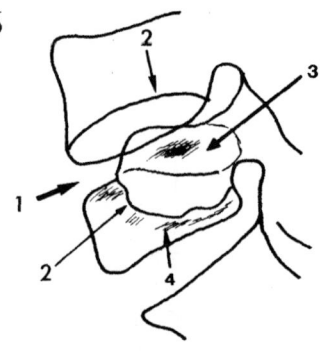 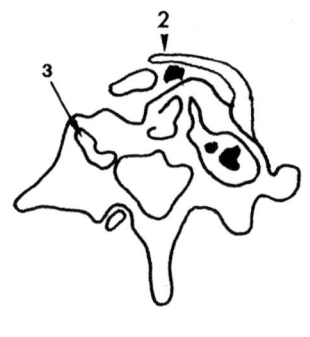

The reader must be able to recognize the presence of four signs:
1 Changes in the intervertebral space.
2 Osteolysis of the cortex of the vertebral bodies adjacent to the intervertebral space.
3 Intracorporeal lytic lesions.
4 Osteosclerosis of the trabecula of bone.
The association of the four signs strongly suggests the diagnosis of vertebral osteomyelitis at L4–L5 interspace.
CT (**c**) permits complete and precise investigation, and shows vertebral lesions, intracanalar extension, and swelling of the adjacent soft tissues.

17

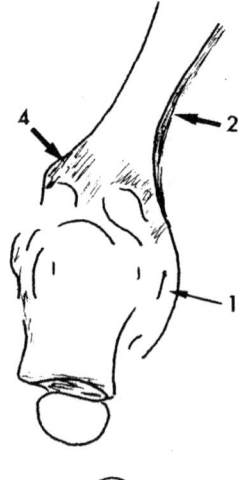

The association of several radiological anomalies:
1 Osteolytic lesions in the femoral and tibial metaphyses,
2 Periosteal bone reactions,
3 Osteoporosis,
4 Limited osteosclerosis,
suggests the diagnosis of malignant hemopathy – lymphoma. These radiological signs are found in about half of the cases. They may be latent, and occur predominantly in the rapid growth areas.

Aneurysmal bone cyst of vertebra.

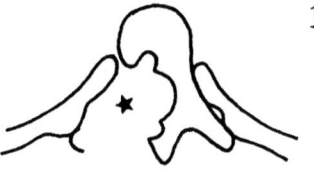

18

A standard radiograph (**a**) shows osteolysis of the right pedicle of T7. Myelography (**b**) confirms the presence of medullary compression in T7. Sagittal tomography (**c**) demonstrates posterior osteolysis at the level of the vertebral body; the anterior limit of the lesion is forwardly convex, with regular and well-defined margins with a thin sclerosis. CT (**d**) confirms the benign nature of the osteolytic lesion, and shows its extension into the posterior soft tissues.

The differential diagnosis is that of an isolated pedicular lysis, and includes osteoblastoma, eosinophil granuloma, a secondary lesion, or lymphoma.

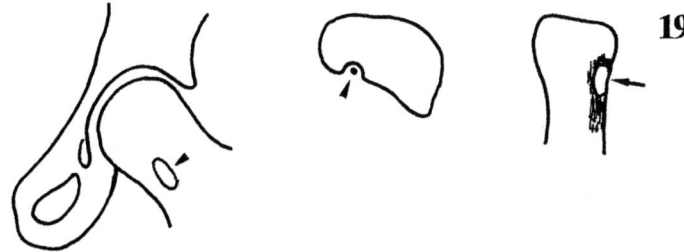

19

Careful study of this radiograph of the pelvis discloses a lucent area in the left femoral neck, without peripheral sclerosis. An axial section CT scan of the left femoral neck (**b**) shows the typical pattern of an osteoid osteoma: a lucent area with peripheral sclerosis, adjacent to the posterior aspect of the left femoral neck, as was proved by the sagittal reconstruction (**c**).

Talonavicular osteo-
arthritis.

1 Loss of articular interspace with irregular articular edges.

2 Subchondral lucent areas and perichondral defects.

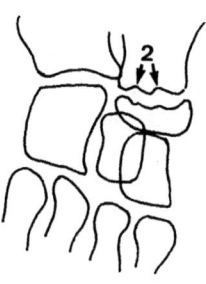
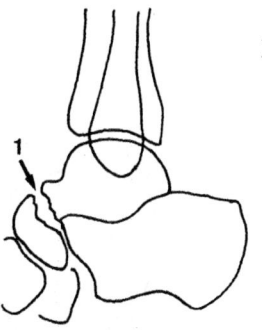

20

Osteoarthritis includes infectious involvement of a joint. Tuberculous osteoarthritis most commonly develops in a chronic manner. Osteoarthritis with trivial organisms usually develops according to an acute pattern.

21

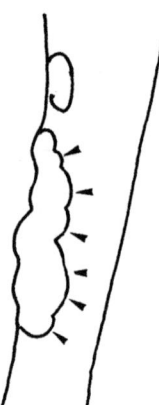

The reader will have readily identified this metaphyseal lesion, which expands the cortex and has a well-defined, serpiginous and sclerotic endosteal margin. It is a *cortical defect.*

22

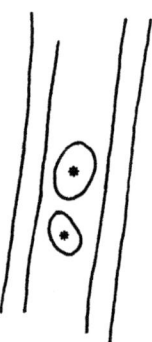

The presence of such lesions with clear-cut margins in the long bones is pathognomonic of myeloma.

23

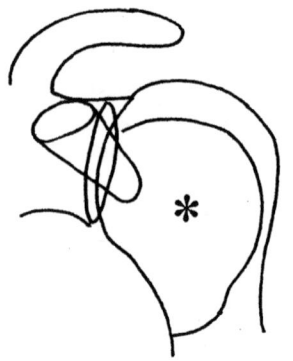

Osteolytic metastasis of the humeral head.

Osteolytic lesion with ill-defined margins, occupying almost the entire humeral head, associated with destruction of the cortex. Arteriography (**b**) shows hypervascularization of a tumoral nature.

Chronic osteomyelitis.

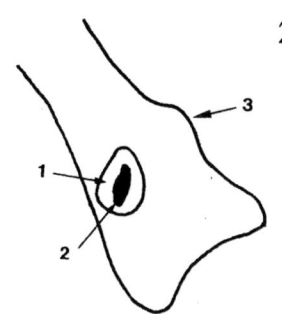

24

1 In the lower extremity of the radius, a lesion surrounded by a sclerotic area.
2 Radiopaque fragment in the center of the lesion.
3 Hypertrophic deformation of the lower extremity of the radius.
4 Signs of radiocarpal arthrosis.

A frontal tomogram (**b**) confirms the presence of an intracavitary sequestrum, reflecting the presence of parcellar bone necrosis. Bacterial contamination of the lower extremity of the radius is secondary to compound fracture and direct inoculation.

Giant cell tumor.

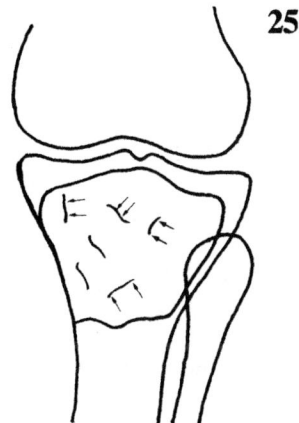

25

Large osteolytic lesion in the epiphysis of the upper end of the tibia. A frontal tomogram (**b**) discloses thin intratumoral septae. This appearance strongly suggests the diagnosis of giant cell tumor.

Aneurysmal bone cyst of the sacrum.

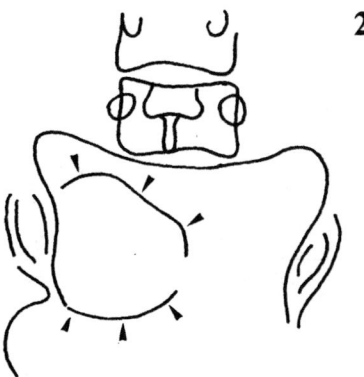

26

Large osteolytic lesion in the sacrum with well-defined borders and discrete peripheral sclerosis (*1*). The adjacent bone structures are unchanged. The overlying soft tissues are not involved. The characteristics of this tumor are better seen on the frontal tomographic section (**b**).

27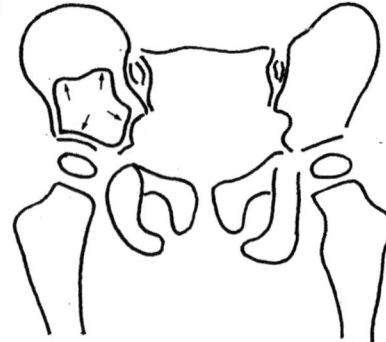

Histiocytosis X.

The routine radiograph of the pelvis shows an osteolytic lesion with well-defined, serpiginous margins and a thin marginal sclerosis. The CT scan provides more details about the lesion: the endosteal aspect of the cortex is eroded, there is a rupture in the continuity of the cortex on the medial aspect of the iliac crest, and there is intratumoral calcification. Histological data are indispensable for making the diagnosis.

28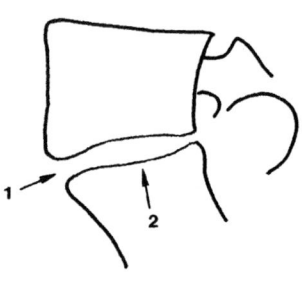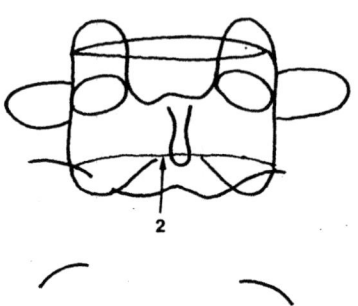

Vertebral osteomyelitis.

Careful study of the radiographs discloses:
- Narrowing of the L5/S1 disk space (*1*).
- The adjacent vertebral plates are demineralized and ill-defined (*2*).

The association of these two signs strongly suggests spondylodiskitis.

29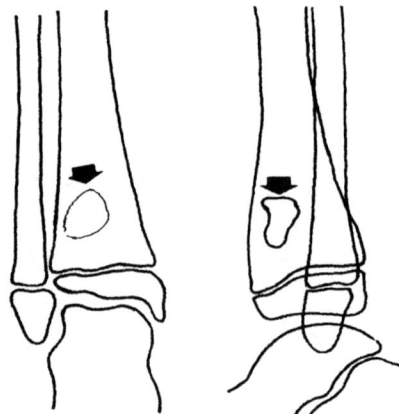

Nonossifying fibroma.

While the diagnosis of the metaphyseal lesion is in doubt from the frontal view, due to indistinct contours, the lateral view shows pathognomonic features of non ossifying fibroma.

Nonossifying fibroma located on the femoral neck.

30

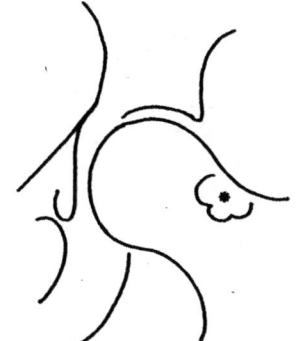

Ewing's sarcoma.

31

1 Extended lytic lesion in the left ischiopubic ramus.
2 Heterogenous condensation of the remaining bone structures of the left ischiopubic ramus.
3 Periosteal reaction.
4 Moderate swelling of the endopelvic soft tissues.

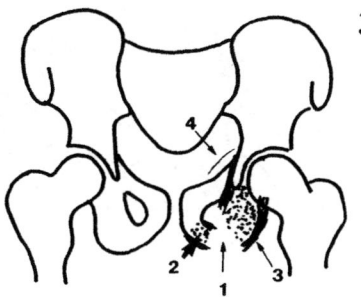

Ewing's sarcoma.

32

1 Heterogeneously increased density of the ischiopubic ramus,
2 periosteal reaction,
3 swelling of the endopelvic soft tissues.

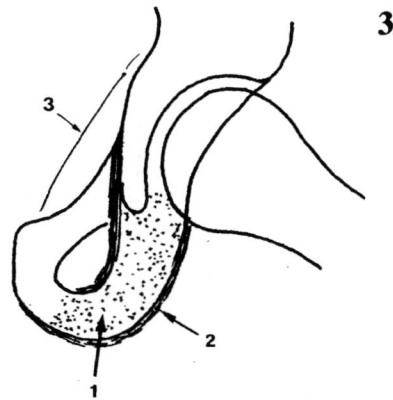

33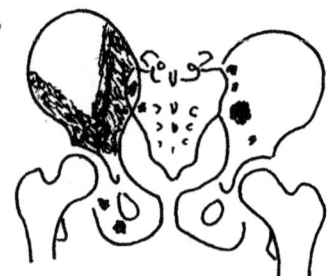

Sclerotic metastases.

Well-defined areas of increased density throughout the pelvis reflect the presence of secondary deposits.

34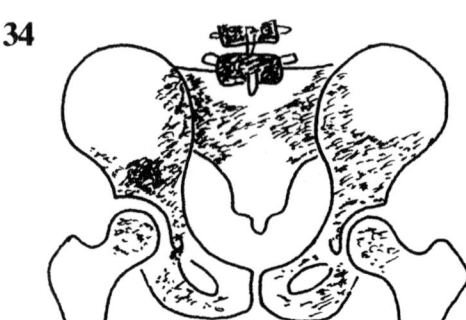

Sclerotic or osteoblastic metastases.

Diffusely increased bone density in the pelvis corresponds to metastatic lesions. The sclerotic pattern is mainly seen in carcinoma of the prostate and of the breast. It may also occur in carcinoma of the lung, of the digestive tract, of the urinary bladder or with hematosarcoma. The most frequent sites for metastatic lesions are the pelvis and the spine.

35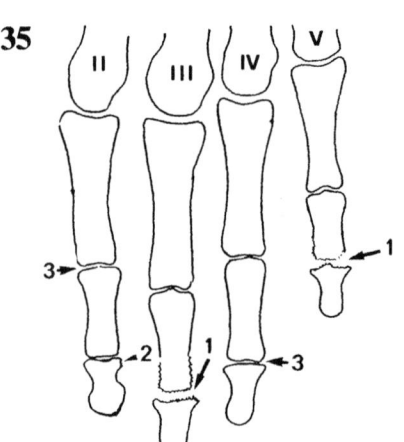

Psoriatic arthritis.

1 Advanced lesions in the distal interphalangeal joints of the third and fifth digits: subchondral erosion, absence of interspace, widening of the articular surfaces, and irregular indistinct periosteal reaction along the diaphyses.
2 Early changes in the distal interphalangeal joint of the second digit, and erosion of the lateral corner of the third phalanx.
3 The interspaces of the proximal and distal interphalangeal joints are narrowed.

Acromegaly.

36

1 Osteophytic hypertrophy of the phalangeal tufts.
2 Distally directed osteophytes on the base of the second phalanx, and broadening of the phalangeal bases.
3 Widened articular space.

These radiological features reflect growth hormone hypersecretion. They are specific to acromegaly.

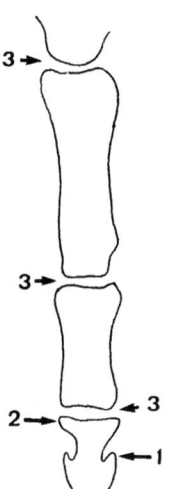

Hypertrophic osteoarthropathy (Marie-Bamberger syndrome).

37

– Periostal new bone formation along the shafts of the metacarpals and phalanges.
– The new bone has smooth contours, variable thickness and undulation of the exterior surface.
– Symetric involvement of the bones is the most frequent finding.

Hypertrophic osteoarthropathy can reveal and is always associated with intrathoracic diseases e. g., chronic pulmonary abscess, benign or malignant tumors of the lungs and thorax. The mecanism is unknown. The lesions usually disappear after removal of the pulmonary neoplasm.

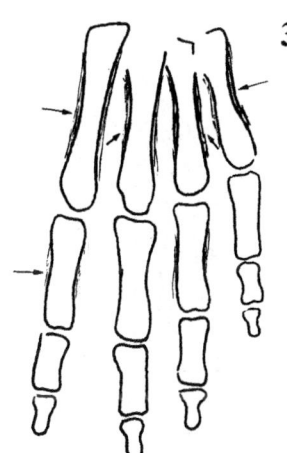

Periostitis of the calcaneus.

38

Erosion and hyperostosis of the posterior surface of the calcaneus at the site of attachment of the Achilles tendon and the plantar fascia. Calcaneitis strongly suggests the presence of ankylosing spondylitis. Uncommonly, it is seen in psoriatic arthritis or in Reiter's syndrome.

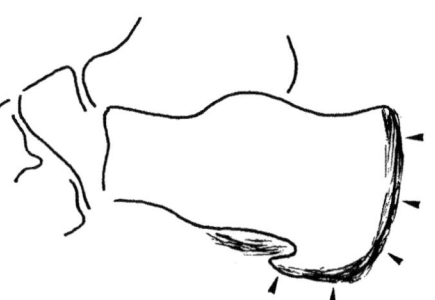

39

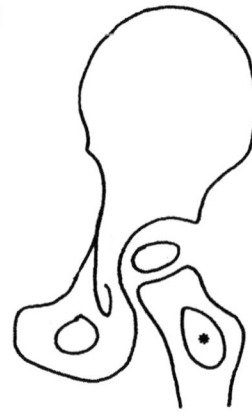

Ewing's sarcoma.

– The routine radiograph (**a**) shows a lucent area with clearly defined margins in the left femoral neck. Note the septae within the lesion.
– A frontal tomogram (**b**) confirms these findings. Compared to a tomograph performed 3 months earlier (**c**), osteolysis is accentuated.
– The CT scan (**d**) reveals an osteolytic lesion adjacent to the anterior aspect of the femoral neck, with destruction of the cortex. The osteolytic lesion shows "saucerisation." The following diagnoses should be discussed: osteomyelitis, osteosarcoma, lymphoma, and histiocytosis X.

40

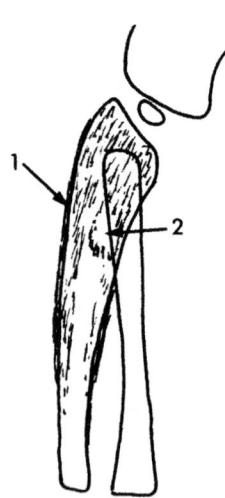

Osteomyelitis.

1 Bone hypertrophy due to periosteal osteophytosis.
2 Two radiolucent areas suggest the presence of abscess cavities.

Physiological "periostitis" of the newborn – a normal variant. **41**

There exist in the newborn, especially the premature, periosteal bone appositions symmetrically distributed along the diaphyses of the long bones. They disappear by the third month.

The main etiologies of "periostitis" in children are:
- Normal variant (newborns)
- Trauma
- Infection: osteomyelitis, congenital syphilis
- Rachitism, scurvy, hypervitaminosis A
- Infantile cortical hyperostosis
- Leukemia and metastases
- Primary bone tumors (Ewing's, osteosarcoma)
- Hemophilia, coagulation disturbances

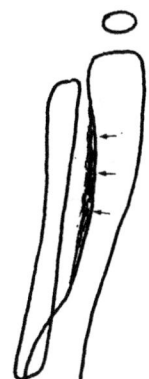

Ewing's sarcoma. **42**

1 Poorly defined heterogeneous, extended osteolysis in the humeral diaphysis.
2 Cortical disruption and lamellar periosteal reaction.
The differential diagnosis is that of osteomyelitis.

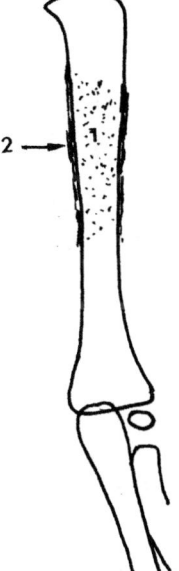

43

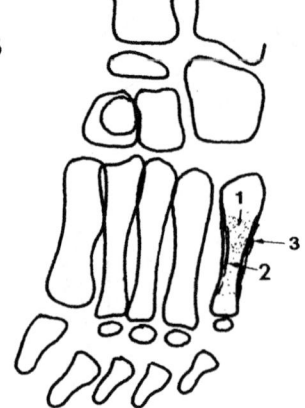

Osteitis of the fifth metatarsal.

Multiple small areas of bone rarefaction, with ill-defined margins; some of them are located in the cortex. Discrete periosteal reaction, lamellar in type.

44

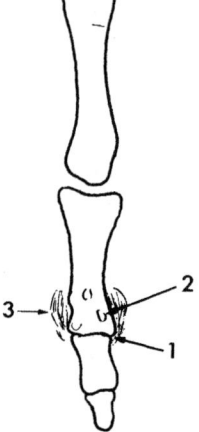

Gout.

1 The articular space of the third proximal metacarpophalangeal joint is narrowed.
2 Subchondral osteolytic areas adjacent to the joint.
3 Swelling of the soft tissues.
The association of these three radiological signs is specific to uratic arthropathy.

45

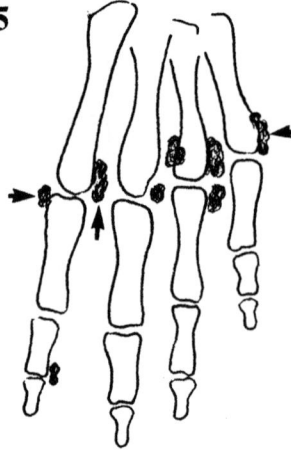

Calcium pyrophosphate deposition disease.

Multiple periarticular calcification, with unchanged articular spaces.

Osteoarthrosis.

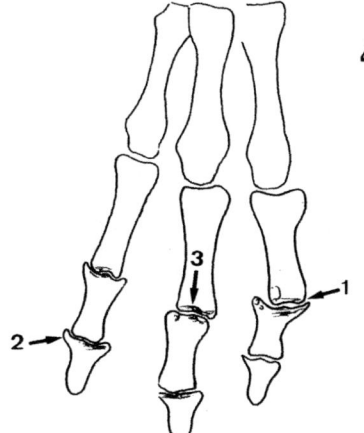

1 Narrowing of the proximal and distal interphalangeal joint spaces.
2 Marginal osteophytosis, causing deformation of the joints.
3 Subchondral sclerosis of the articular surfaces.

Cyst of the calcaneus.

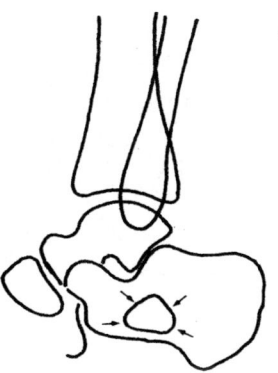

Clearly delineated homogeneous lucent area.

Sessile osteochondroma.

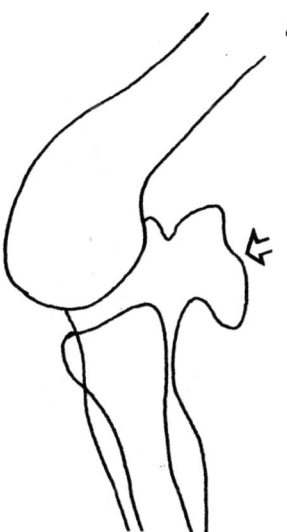

Exostosis with a large base developing on the coronoid process of the ulna. Note its cupula-shaped image on the anterior surface of the humeral metaphysis.

49

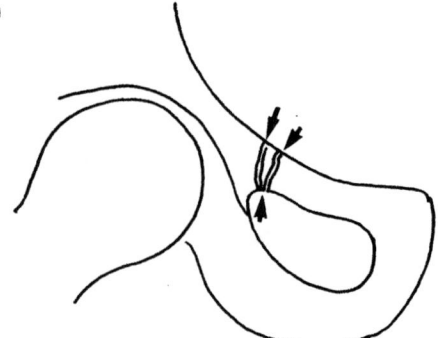

Stress fracture of the iliopubic ramus.

Increased radiolucency of the bone. Disruption in the continuity of the iliopubic ramus without evidence of a callus. Subchondral sclerosis of the fracture edges.

50

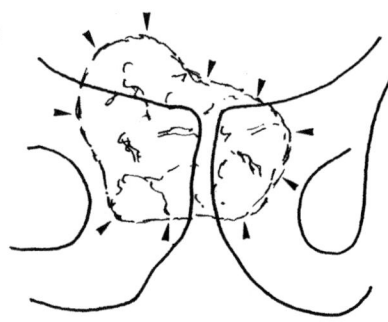

Osteochondroma.

Polylobular radiolucent area, delineated by a sclerotic line. Presence of calcification, and "soapbubble" appearance.

51

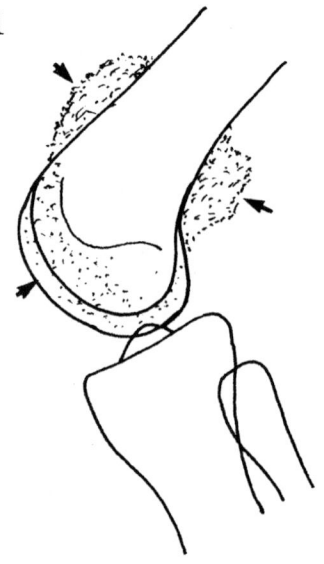

Osteosarcoma of the distal end of the femur.

Heterogeneous osteolysis in the distal end of the femur, with cortical disruption, and extension to the soft tissues. Arteriography (**c**) confirms the malignant nature of the tumor, and shows marked anarchic neovascularization.

Chondrosarcoma of vertebra.

Large tumoral lesion developing from the left posterior hemiarch of L2. Extension to the adjacent soft tissues, containing anarchic calcification. CT scanning demonstrates the intracanalar extension of the tumor, and provides greater detail about invasion of the soft tissues.

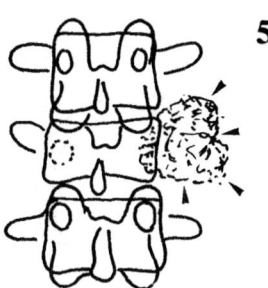

52

Osteosarcoma of the distal end of the femur.

Ill-defined, patchy osteolysis associated with disruption of the cortex (*1*). Lamellar periosteal reaction on the anterior surface of the femur (*2*), and spicular reaction on the posterior surface (*3*). These features are demonstrated in even greater detail on the CT scan (**c**).

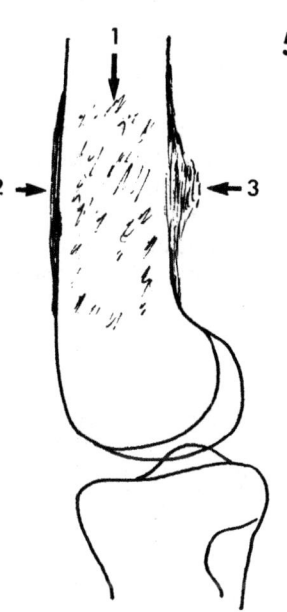

53

54

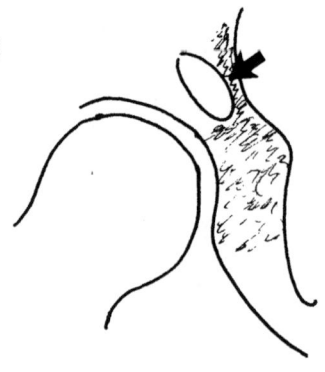 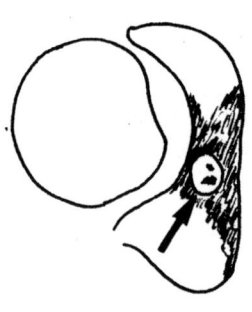

Osteoid osteoma in the right acetabulum.

Well-defined lesion surrounded by sclerosis in the deepest part of the right acetabulum.

The acetabulum is deformed. Tomograms (**c**) provides more details about the lesion. CT axial sections (**d**) and sagittal reconstruction (**e**) demonstrate the presence of a well-defined lesion with central calcification, and surrounding reactive sclerosis.

These features strongly suggest the diagnosis of osteoid osteoma. Note the moderate enlargement of the articular space, reflecting intra-articular effusion due to lymphofollicular synovitis.

55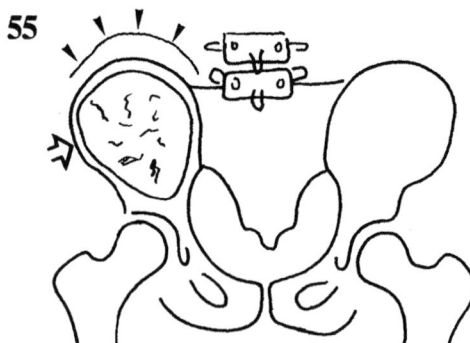

Ewing's sarcoma.

Heterogeneous, ill-defined, and diffuse osteolysis in the upper part of the right ilium. Extension to the adjacent soft tissues is evidenced by an opacity overlapping the upper pole of the ilium. CT scanning (**c**) confirms the extension into the soft tissues, and demonstrates the degree of osteolysis.

56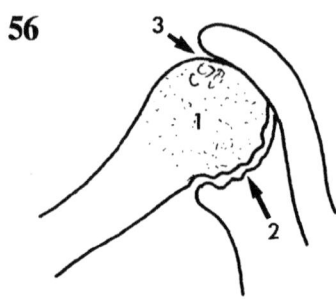

Rheumatoid arthritis.

1 Increased radiolucency of the humeral head.
2 Global narrowing of the glenohumeral joint space with "festooned" appearance of the articular surfaces of the humeral head and glenoid cavity.
3 Atrophic remodelling of the superior aspect of the greater tubercle, with elevation of the humeral head.

Rheumatoid arthritis.

1 Regional osteoporosis.
2 Absence of glenohumeral joint space.
3 Erosions on the superior aspect of the humeral head.
4 Elevation of the humeral head, and subacromial sclerosis.

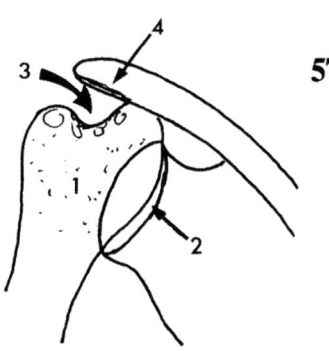

57

Rheumatoid arthritis.

Erosion of the superolateral part of the humeral head with subjacent lucent lesions; narrowing of the glenohumeral space; elevation of the humeral head.

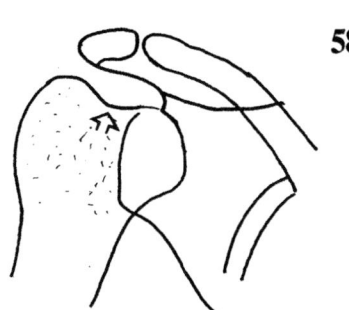

58

Osteolytic metastasis.

Ill-defined extended osteolysis of the glenoid cavity and of the neck of the scapula. Note the rounded, radiolucent lesion on the greater tubercle of the humerus. This is a normal variant, to be differentiated from a metastasis.

59

Calcinosis.

Periarticular polycyclic calcic deposits.
Calcinosis is a condition characterized by the presence of calcification in the subcutaneous connective, deep perimuscular, peritendinous, and periarticular tissues. In 40% of cases, calcinosis is seen in collagen vascular diseases, such as dermatomyositis and scleroderma. Soft tissue calcification can be produced by other systemic diseases (metabolic or vascular diseases, infestations, infections, arthritides) or local phenomena, such as trauma or local destruction.

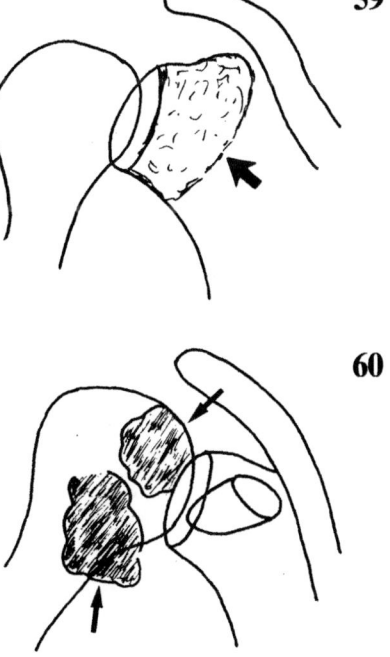

60

61

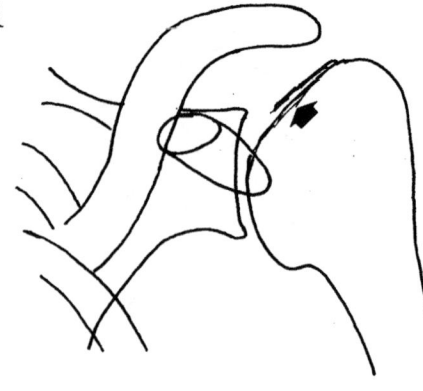

Aseptic necrosis of the humeral head.

Depression in the superolateral part of the humeral head, caused by fracture of the subchondral bone. Collapse of the head is delayed. The glenohumeral joint space is unchanged.
Remodelling of the bone structure. Aseptic necrosis of the humeral head is seldom idiopathic. It is usually secondary to corticosteroid therapy, Gaucher's disease, drepanocytosis, or dysbaric conditions (caisson disease).

62

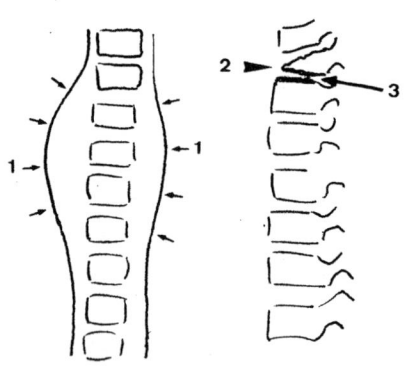

T5/6 spondylitis.

1 Voluminous paravertebral spindle. Changes in the paravertebral soft tissues reflect the presence of an abscess causing backward displacement of the paraspinal lines.
2 Wedge compression of the vertebral body of T5.
3 Narrowing of the T5/6 disk space.
4 Disturbed spinal static curvature, and loss of physiologic curvature.

Differential diagnosis of changes in the paravertebral lines:
- Osteomyelitis of spine with abscess,
- Spontaneous or idiopathic hematoma,
- Metastatic neoplasm,
- Lymphoma,
- Myeloma,
- Osteophytosis,
- Aneurysm or unfolding of the aorta,
- Neurogenic tumor.

Narvopathic calcification

Bilateral ossification of the glutei, with pericapsular bone appositions. Nervous paraosteoarthropathies are seen after longstanding immobilization due to such conditions as: paralysis, hemiplegia, coma, major burns, tetanus.

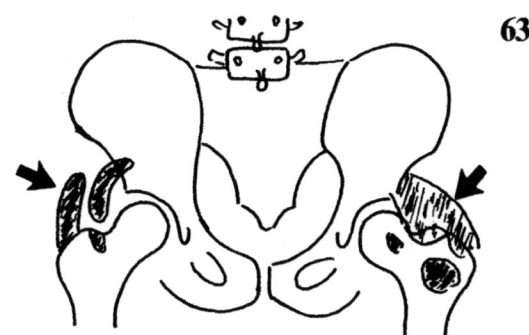

63

Idiopathic ischemic necrosis (femoral head).

A comparative study of the two hips shows:
1 The left femoral head has lost its spherical shape.
2 Superolateral area of osteocondensation, corresponding to necrosis.
3 Clear subchondral line ("egg-shell" image).
4 Normal joint space and condyle.
These features permit the diagnosis of the onset of ischemic osteonecrosis.

64

Scaphoidotrapezial arthrosis and rhizarthrosis.

Narrowed articular space, subchondral sclerosis, and osteophytosis of the margins in the scaphoidotrapezial and trapezometacarpal articulations of the thumb.

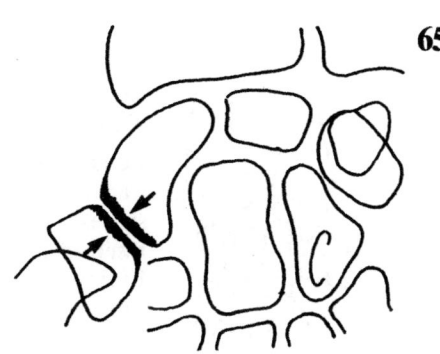

65

66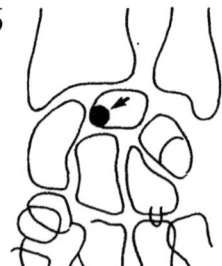

Bone island in the lunate.

Well-defined, rounded, homogeneous condensation area. This asymptomatic lesion without pathological significance is a normal variant.

67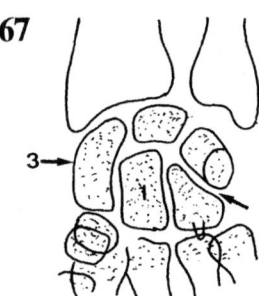

Sudeck's atrophy.

- Heterogeneous, irregular osteoporosis of the carpal bones. This appearance signals the development of the disease.
- Uninvolved articular spaces. This characteristic is necessary to affirm the diagnosis.
- The bone contours are well delineated and unaffected.

These signs are detected from comparative films (compare with the normal appearance). The radiological manifestations can be retarded by 3–4 weeks. Their location is usually segmental – hand, wrist, shoulder.

68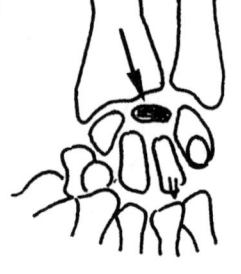

Ischemic necrosis (carpal semilunar);
Kienböck's disease.

Condensation of the lunate, which is crushed and fragmented. The other carpal bones and the articular spaces are unaffected. Osteonecrosis is usually the result of major trauma or of repeated microtrauma. Later on, radiocarpal arthrosis develops. Treatment is surgical, with prosthetic replacement of the joint.

Right sacroiliitis.

A comparative study of both sacroiliac joints shows anomalies on the right side:
– Widening of the articular space.
– Indistinct and irregular articular edges.
– Regional osteoporosis.
Frontal tomogram (**b**) confirms the diagnosis. Unilateral sacroiliitis is probably due to localized infection.

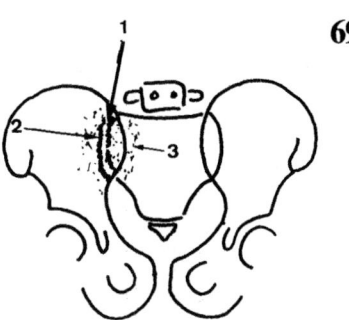

69

Osteolytic metastasis of the axis.

The sagittal tomogram shows a marked osteolytic lesion with ill-defined margins in the body of the axis. The odontoid process is uninvolved. The finding of such lesions at a prefractural stage permits preventive treatment with surgery or radiotherapy.

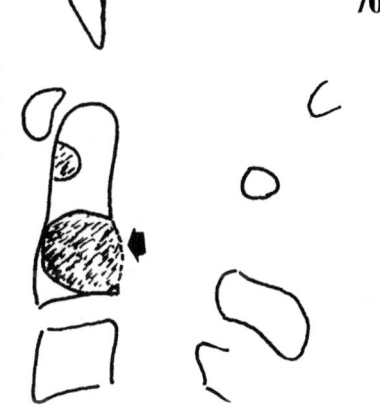

70

Osteolytic metastasis of the atlas.

Axial section of CT scan shows lysis in the right lateral mass and right anterior hemiarch. The odontoid process is displaced to the right, signifying the rupture of the transverse ligament.

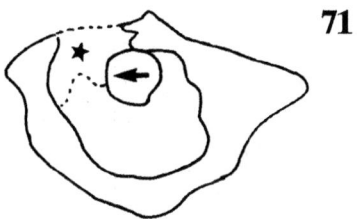

71

72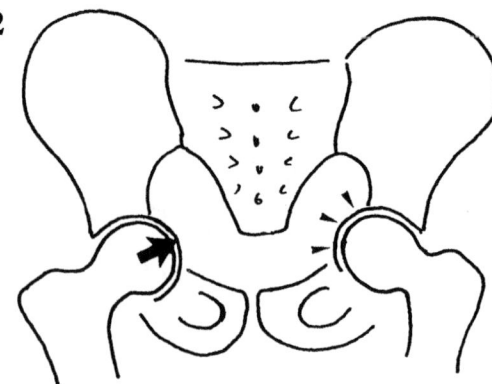

Protrusive osteoarthritis of the hip.

The hip joints tend to protrude into the pelvic cavity. This condition is consistent with acetabular protrusion; in the present case it is bilateral. This is a case of secondary osteoarthritis of the hip, of the medial pattern. The joint space is narrowed in its inferior part, and normal in its superior part.

73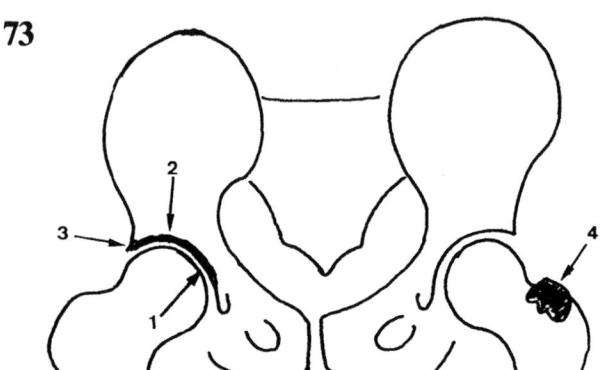

Initial stage of osteoarthritis of the hip.

1 Superomedial narrowing of the right joint space. This type is less common than superior or lateral narrowing.
2 Subchondral condensation of the acetabulum.
3 Onset of osteophytosis on the acetabulum and femoral head.
Note the presence of calcifying periarthritis of the left hip – calcification in the neighborhood of the greater trochanter (*4*).

74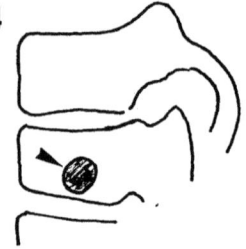

Sclerotic metastasis of a vertebra.

Rounded, homogeneous opacity with ill-defined contours in the vertebral body. The differential diagnosis of this single osteoblastic localization is the benign condensing focus. The sclerotic reaction adjacent to the metastasis is responsible for the osteoblastic condensing lesion. Such lesions are frequently multiple and scattered throughout the bone.

Osteolytic vertebral metastases.

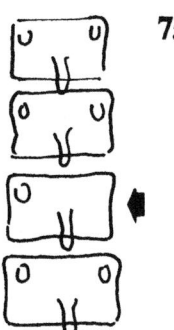

75

– Diffuse vertebral osteoporosis with compression of the vertebrae,
– hazy appearance, and poor visualization of the left pedicles of T10 and T11.
– The left pedicle of T9 is not visible.
– The left paravertebral line is displaced laterally.
Bone resorption adjacent to the metastasis has caused the formation of cavities which render the bone fragile. Extension of osteolysis causes cortical disruption, spontaneous fracture, or expansion into the soft tissues.

Sclerotic vertebral metastasis.

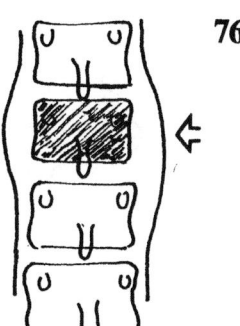

76

Global condensation of the vertebral body and of the pedicles of T8, without deformation. Compare with the normal appearance of the superior and inferior vertebrae. The disk space height is unchanged. The paravertebral mediastinal lines are displaced and delineate a paravertebral spindle.

Ankylosing spondylitis.

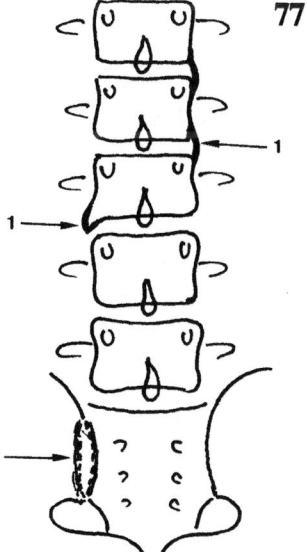

77

1 The presence of syndesmophytes: infraligamentous ossifications, extending vertically from one vertebra to the other, delineate the disc contours.
2 Bilateral sacroiliac ankylosis and absence of articular spaces.
These are two signs specific to ankylosing spondylitis
– chronic inflammatory rheumatism mainly affecting the spine and the pelvis, with a tendency toward ankylosis. Ankylosing spondylitis mainly affects young adult males.

78

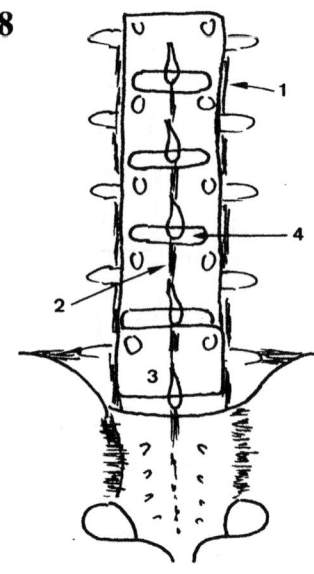

Ankylosing spondylitis evolves with acute episodes and intermittent remission periods. Stiffness develops, ascending from the pelvis to the cervical spine.

1 Infraligamentous ossifications involving the entire spine duplicate the contours of the intervertebral discs, and are responsible for the typical "bamboo spine" appearance.
2 Ossification of the interspinous and yellow ligaments produces vertical and parallel ossification lines, responsible for the "trolley-track" sign.
3 Diffuse osteoporosis.
4 The vertebral bodies and the intervertebral disc spaces are unchanged.

79

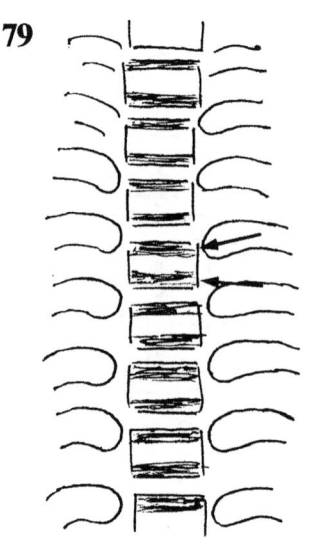

Osteopetrosis.

Osteocondensation bands adjacent to, and parallel to the vertebral plates, responsible for the "sandwich" appearance, strongly suggest the diagnosis of osteopetrosis – genotypic osteopathy, with increased bone density resulting from a decrease in the rate of bone and cartilage resorption.

Osteolytic metastasis of the cortex.

– The frontal projection (**a**) shows an oval lesion with a vertical long axis and clearly defined margins. There is periosteal reaction.
– The lateral projection (**b**) shows osteolysis of the cortex without involvement of the soft tissues.
– Axial CT provides accurate visualization of the lesion: destruction localized to the cortex with intramedullary extension and involvement of the adjacent soft parts (**c**).

80

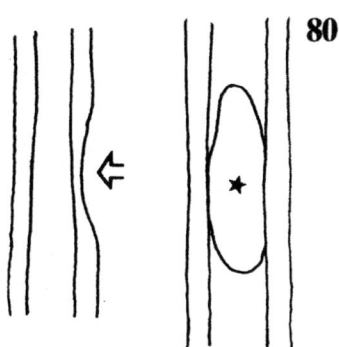

Psoriatic rheumatism.

1 Destructive lesions of the lacunar type, with clearly defined margins, located on the distal end of the radius and of the ulna, and on the scaphoid.
2 Changes in the carpometacarpal joints at the level of the capitate, the trapezium and the trapezoid – hazy appearance and irregular articular edges.

81

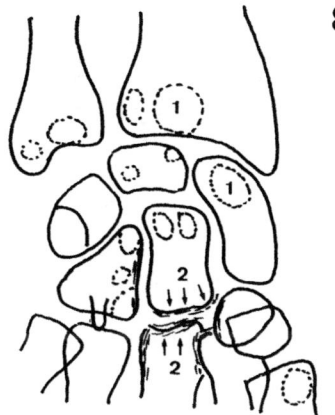

Radiocarpal arthritis.

1 Osteoporosis confined to the bone segments adjacent to the radiocarpal joint.
2 Widened joint space.
3 Irregular articular edges with signs of erosion.
4 Erosions in the distal end of the radius, in the scaphoid and in the lunate.

This appearance corresponds to advanced arthritis.

82

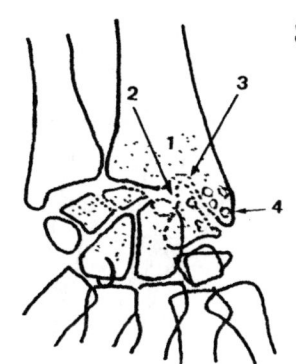

83

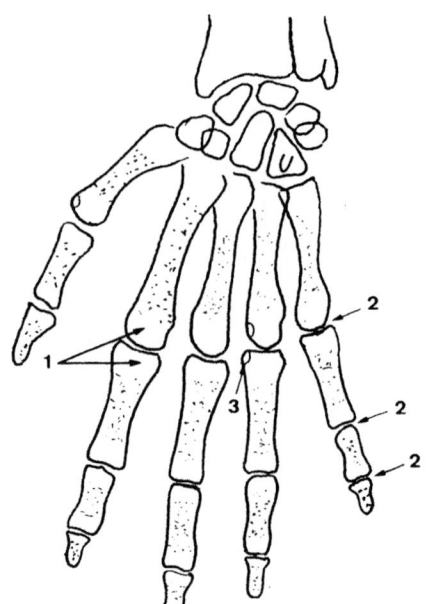

Rheumatoid arthritis.

The association of the following features, which are neither early in onset, nor specific, must suggest the diagnosis of rheumatoid arthritis:
1 Band-shaped demineralization on either side of the metacarpophalangeal and interphalangeal joints.
2 Loss of joint space.
3 Erosions in the phalangeal ends.
4 Swelling of the soft tissues around the metacarpophalangeal and interphalangeal joints.

84

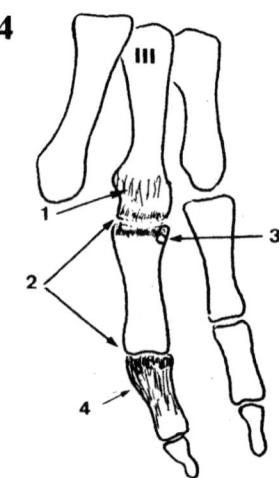

Arthritis of the metacarpophalangeal and interphalangeal joints on the third finger.

1 Heterogeneously increased density in the third metacarpal, the first and the second phalanges.
2 Joint space narrowing in the metacarpophalangeal, proximal and distal interphalangeal joints.
3 Subchondral erosions in the third metacarpal head, the extremities of the first and second phalanx and in the base of the distal phalanx.
4 The metacarpal and phalanges are deformed by periosteal reaction.

Rheumatoid arthritis.

1 Joint space narrowing in the metacarpophalangeal joints of the second and third fingers, as well as in the proximal interphalangeal joints.

2 Distal interphalangeal subluxations.

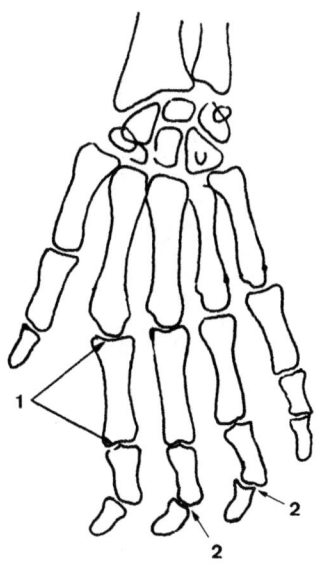

Rheumatoid arthritis.

– Narrowing of the joint spaces in the carpus: the appearance is that of carpitis.
– Metacarpophalangeal, proximal and distal interphalangeal arthritis.
– Erosions in the metacarpal heads and in the phalanges.
– Cysts in the radial and ulnar extremities.
– Osteoporosis.

This appearance reflects advanced rheumatoid arthritis.

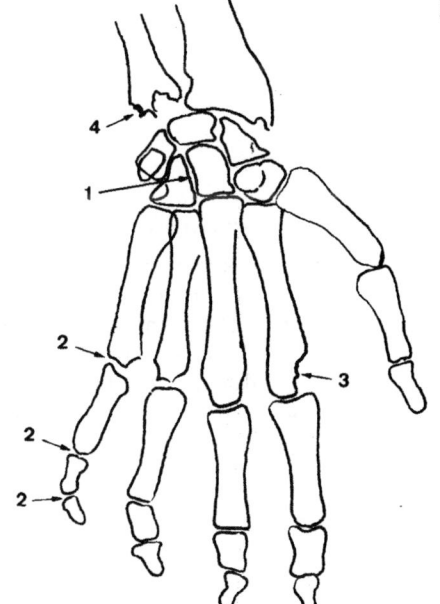

87

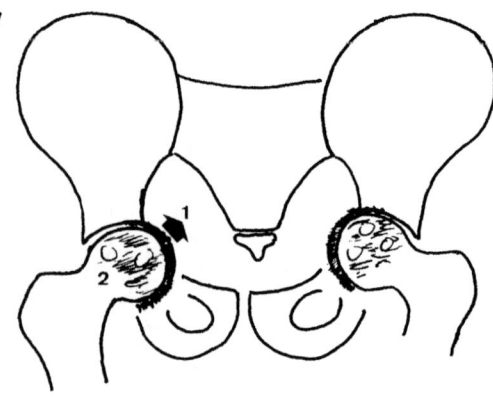

Protrusive osteoarthritis of the hip.

- Evident acetabular protrusion (*1*).
- Both femoral heads show the characteristics of advanced arthritis: obliteration of the joint space, osteophytosis, subchondral sclerosis, and cysts (*2*).

88

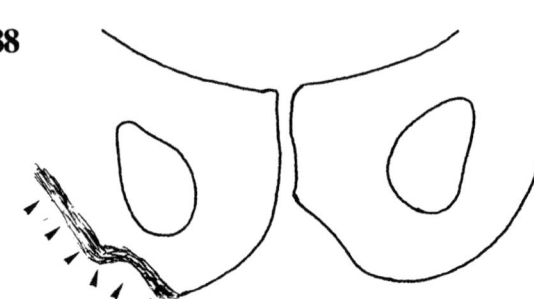

Osteitis of the right ischium.

Erosions with ill-defined margins in the right ischial tuberosity. Compare this with the normal appearance of the left ischium.

89

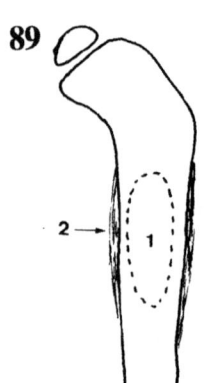

Osteomyelitis of the femur.

1 Radiolucent area surrounded by discrete sclerosis in the femoral diaphysis.
2 Deformation of the diaphysis of widening type, due to periosteal reaction.

Together with the clinical and biological data, these radiological features suggest the diagnosis of osteomyelitis.

Osteolytic metastasis.

The frontal projection (**a**) reveals an eccentric lucent area with indistinct margins and associated periosteal reaction.
The lateral projection (**b**) shows erosion of the cortex. Expansion into the soft tissues is delineated by a thin calcic shell (*arrows*) of periosteal origin. Periosteal lysis is responsible for spur formations (*arrowheads*).

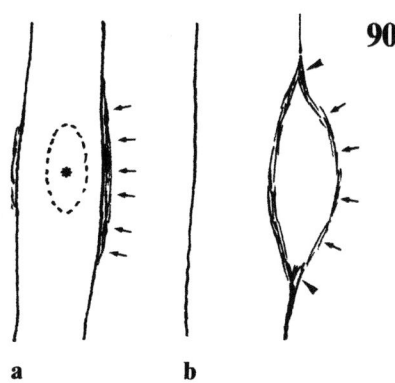

90

a   **b**

Osteoid osteoma.

Marked localized and homogeneous thickening of the cortex, containing a small lucent area. This appearance strongly suggests the diagnosis of osteoid osteoma. This is reinforced by radionuclide scanning, which shows unusually early increased uptake of the tracer in this area.
A localized chronic osteomyelitis may sometimes present an identical appearance.

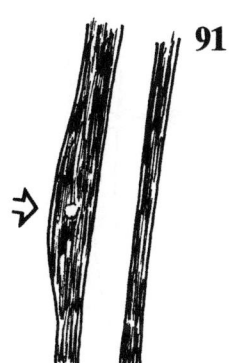

91

Post-traumatic osteoma.

Routine radiographs (**a**), as well as the CT scan (**b**) reveal calcification of the soft tissues in the neighborhood of the bone, but clearly distinct from it – post-traumatic calcification.
Post-traumatic hematomas may calcify and secondarily become osseous. Initially, the calcification has a low density. Later, the density increases and the margins are better defined. When there is no history of trauma, the differential diagnosis is that of parosteal or juxtacortical sarcoma.
CT is very helpful in showing the connections of the calcified mass with the adjacent bone.

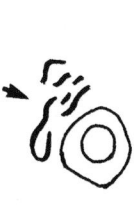

92

93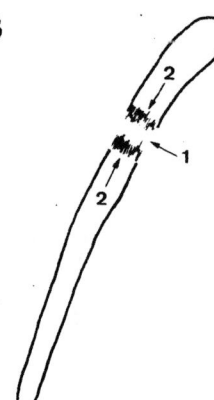

Manubriosternal arthritis.

The radiological features of arthritis are present in the manubriosternal joint:

1 Widening of the joint space.
2 Hazy appearance of the articular edges, with destruction of cortex and subchondral erosions.
3 The pre- and retrosternal soft tissues are not yet significantly altered.

All these features are shown in greater detail on a midsagittal tomogram (**b**).

94

Osteitis of the sternal manubrium.

The radiological features of chronic osteomyelitis are present in the sternal manubrium:

1 Bone hypertrophy following subperiosteal osteophytosis.
2 Irregular opacity of the manubrium.
3 Presence of radiolucent areas.

95

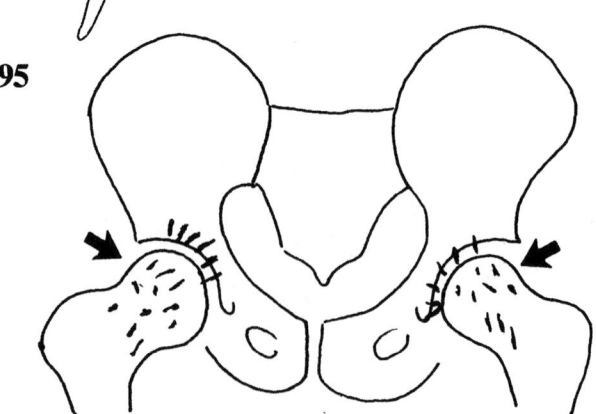

Osteopoikilosis (striated form).

Opaque striations in the acetabulum, the femoral ends and the pubic symphysis. Osteopoikilosis is a dystrophic condition characterized by the presence of small, spicular or rounded condensations distributed over the epiphyses of the hands and feet and in the spongy bone of the pelvis and scapulae.

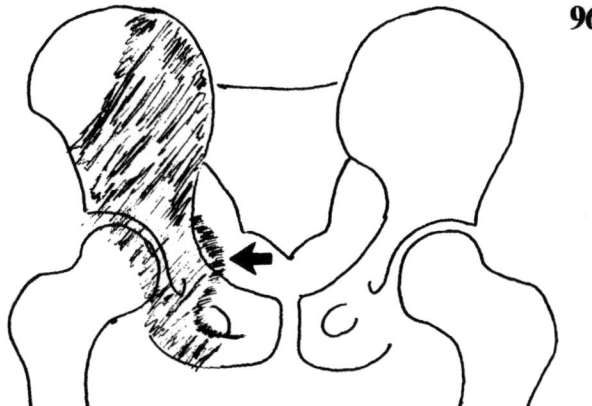

Sarcomatous degeneration in Paget's disease.

Diffuse condensation of the left hemipelvis with spiculations characteristic of osteosarcoma. Hypertrophy and coarsened structure of the femoral head, the iliopubic and ilioischial rami indicate the pagetic involvement.

Vertebral block – a sequel of spondylitis.

Deformation of the thoracic spine due to the destruction of two vertebral bodies. This appearance is a consequence of the spondylodiskitis, of which several signs persist:
1 Absence of joint space,
2 cortical osteolysis,
3 paradiscal erosion.
There are also signs of repair with the formation of a kyphotic vertebral block responsible for the gibbosity. Note the presence of a subjacent congenital vertebral block with persistence of a space between the two vertebrae.

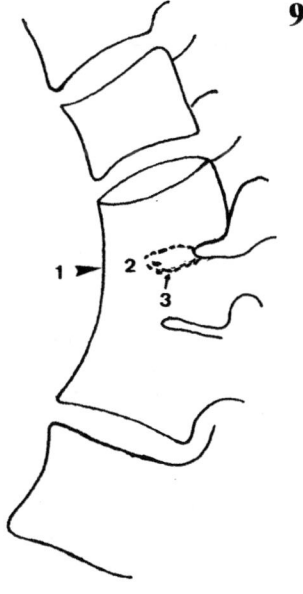

98

Osteolytic metastasis of T12.

1 Deformation and marked compression of the vertebral body.
2 Destroyed cortex.
3 Osteolytic foci in the vertebral body.

99

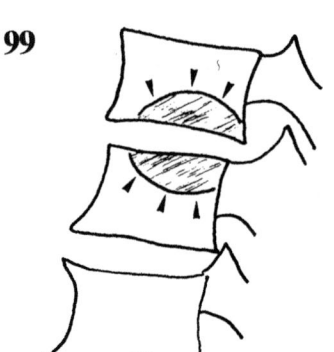

Osteoarthritis of the lumbar spine.

Semicircular opacities adjacent to several intervertebral disk spaces correspond to the projection in the sagittal plane of huge lateral osteophytes.

100

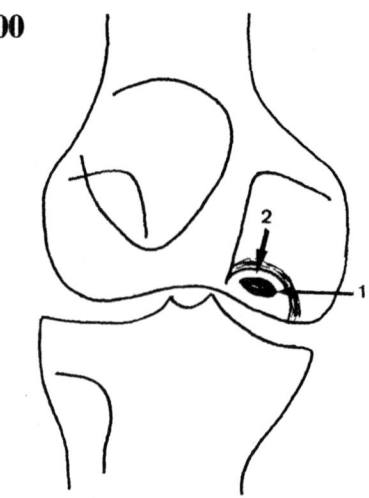

Osteochondritis dissecans of the medial femoral condyle.

Dense bone fragment (*1*) separated from the bone by a clear line (*2*). This fragment may become loose, and is thus liable to cause blocking of the joint.

Acromegaly; Erdheim spondylosis.

101

1 Ankylosing spondyloarthritis of all vertebral bodies.

2 Prevertebral subperiosteal bone deposition increases the anteroposterior diameters of the vertebral bodies.

3 Multilevelled diskarthrosis.

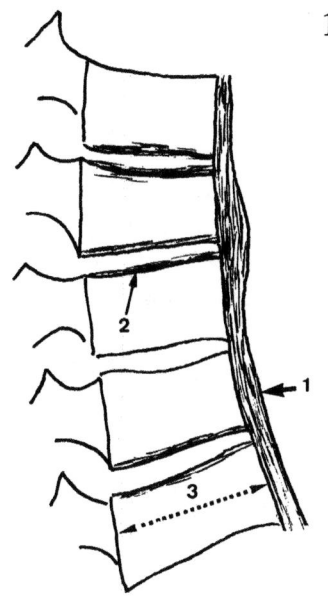

Sarcoidosis.

102

All types of bone lesions occurring in sarcoidosis are seen on this radiograph of the hand:

1 Erosions and marginal erosions with destruction of the distal phalanx of the fourth finger.

2 Erosions and marginal erosions in the first phalanx of the second and fifth fingers.

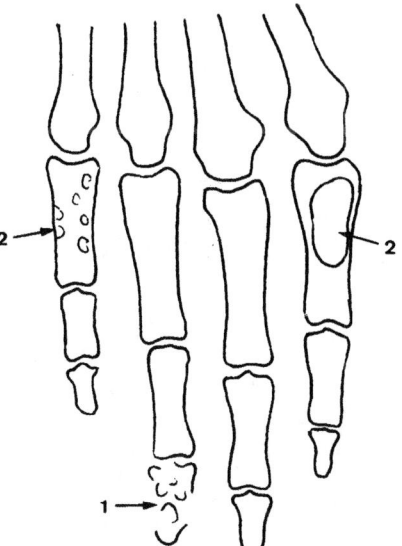

139

103

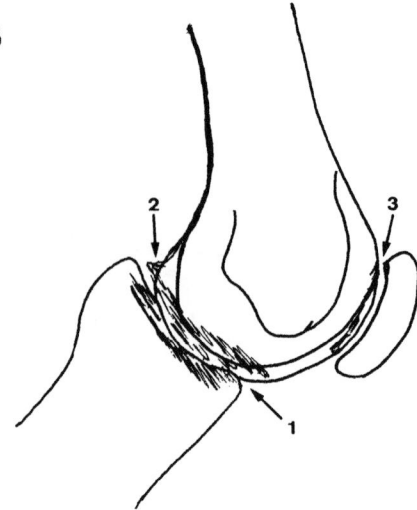

Osteoarthritis of the knee.

1 Obliteration of the femorotibial interspace, with subchondral sclerosis.
2 Femorotibial osteophytosis.
3 Osteoarthritis of the patellofemoral compartment and joint space narrowing.
Moderate subchondral osteosclerosis and patellar osteophytosis. Abnormal relations between the patella and the trochlea contribute to the development of patellofemoral osteoarthritis.

104

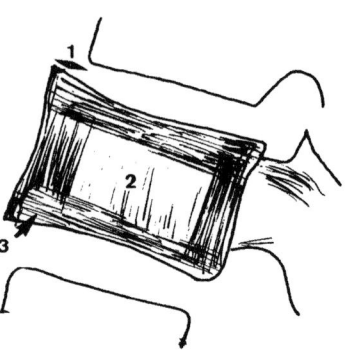

Vertebra in Paget's disease.

1 Hypertrophic vertebral body – increase of anteroposterior diameter.
2 Coarsening of the bone structure.
3 "Picture frame" vertebral body.
The association of these three signs is pathognomonic of Paget's disease. Note also the hypertrophy and the coarsened trabeculae in the pedicles.

105

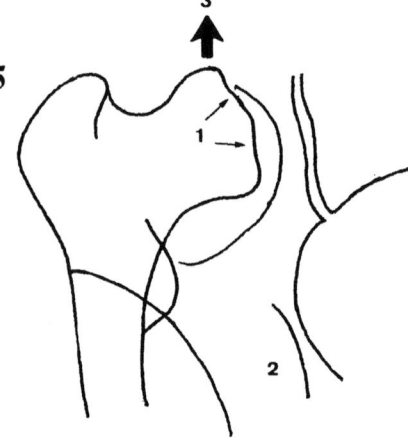

Dislocation of the hip.

1 The femoral head is irregular and flattened.
2 Hypoplastic acetabulum.
3 Abnormally high femoral head.
This is an inveterate dislocation of the hip in a case of congenital dysplasia of the hip.

Leukemia.

Presence of lucent bands in the metaphyses of the femoral ends. The diagnosis depends on the child's age: in children over 18 months, one thinks mainly of a malignant hemopathy, or of metastases from a neuroblastoma. The presence of lucent bands in the metaphyses should lead one to perform a blood cell count and a myelogram.

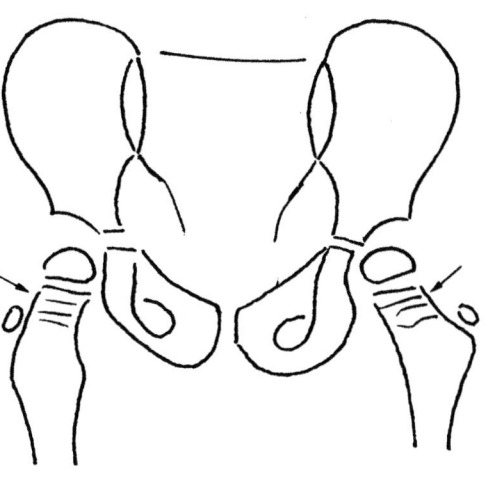

The etiology of radiolucent metaphyseal bands includes:
- Normal variant
- Neonatal stress
- Embryofetopathy (toxoplasmosis, rubella, syphilis etc.)
- Leukemia,
- Metastases (neuroblastoma)
- Cushing's syndrome
- Hypervitaminosis D
- Osteogenesis imperfecta.

Osteoporosis.

1 Diffuse increase of the spinal radiolucency.
2 Biconcave appearance of the vertebral bodies.
3 The vertebral cortex is thin, well-defined and continuous.
4 Interspinous arthrosis: Baastrup's disease.

The radiological syndrome of osteoporosis has different etiologies: senile, postmenopausal, steroid-induced.

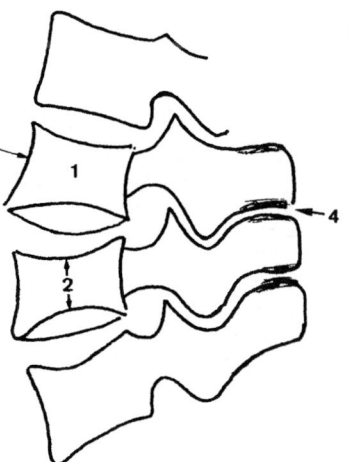

108

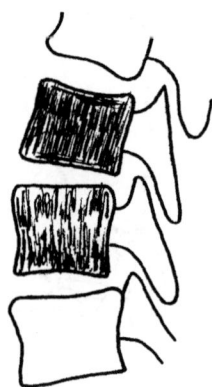

Myeloid metaplasia.

1 Diffuse increase in vertebral bone density,
2 Hypertrophied vertical trabeculations,
3 Absence of vertebral deformation.
Myelofibrosis mainly affects sites of active hematopoiesis, for example, pelvis, vertebrae, sternum, and ribs.

109

Diffuse sclerotic metastases.

– Diffuse increase in vertebral density,
– Absence of coarsening,
– Absence of morphological changes in the bone segments.

110

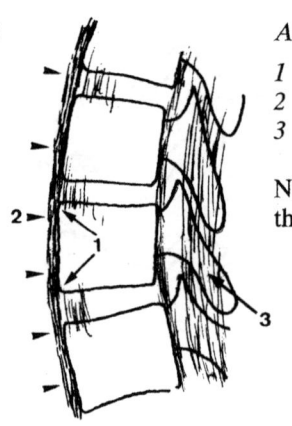

Ankylosing spondylitis.

1 The vertebral bodies have a square appearance.
2 Their anterior aspects are united by bony bridges.
3 Ligamentous ossification also unites the articular processes.
Note the presence of a benign condensation focus in the body of L1.

Ankylosing spondylitis.

Vertebral squaring, with onset of intervertebral bone bridges: onset of syndesmophytes. This is an early stage of ankylosing spondylitis.

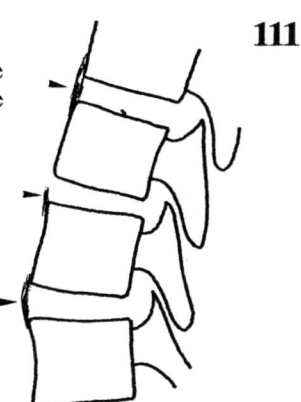

111

Fracture of a vertebra in ankylosing spondylitis.

Subligamentous ossification on the anterior aspect of the vertebral bodies, and presence of syndesmophytes allows to diagnose ankylosing spondylitis. Fracture of the L2 vertebral body is a complication, due to ankylosis of the spine.

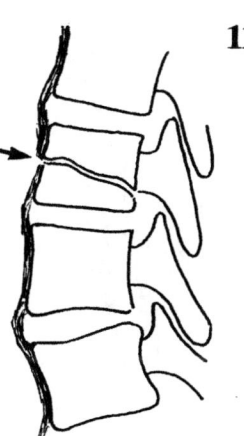

112

Calcific periarthritis of the hip.

Calcific deposits over the greater trochanter.

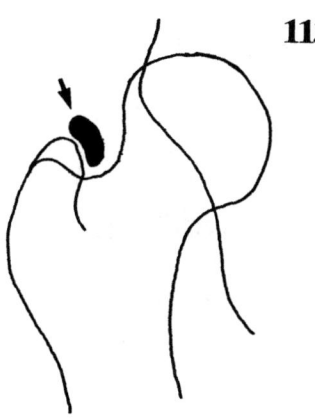

113

114

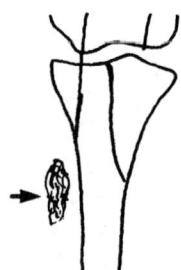

Post-traumatic osteoma.

Calcification of the periosseous soft tissues, corresponding to a calcified hematoma.

115

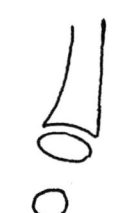

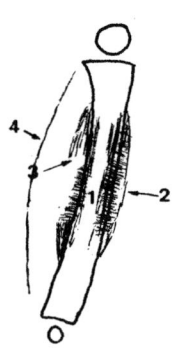

Ewing's sarcoma.

1 Lytic lesion in the left tibial diaphysis, with sclerosis of the involved bone.
2 Spicular and lamellar periosteal reactions.
3 Periosteal disruption with Codmann spur.
4 Extension to the soft tissues.

116

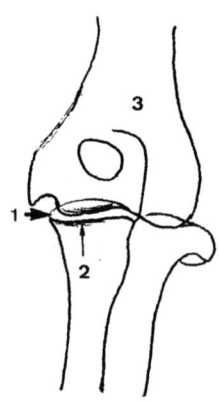

Rheumatoid polyarthritis.

1 Joint space narrowing.
2 Subchondral erosions.
3 The radiolucency of the bone segments is increased.
These features are characteristic of rheumatic arthritis and, primarily, of rheumatoid polyarthritis.

Synovial osteochondromatosis.

1 The bone segments are neither deformed nor altered.
2 The articular space is only slightly modified, with signs of the onset of arthropathy.
3 Heterogeneous, calcified, oval opacity at the level of the epicondyle. This opacity reflects the presence of a foreign body; its intra-articular location can be confirmed by arthrography.

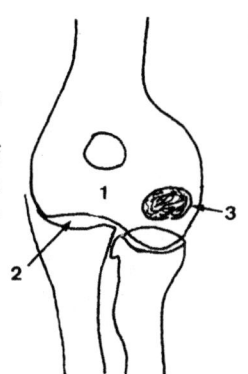

117

Rheumatoid arthritis.

Marked destruction and displacement of the axis of the bones correspond to an advanced stage of the inflammatory disease.

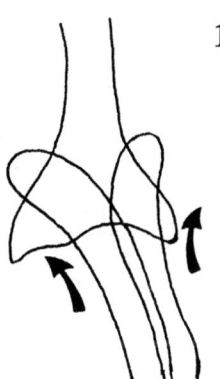

118

Articular chondrocalcinosis.

The presence of a calcic line in the triangular fibrocartilage and the different articular spaces of the carpus reflect calcium pyrophosphate dihydrate crystal deposition in the cartilage.

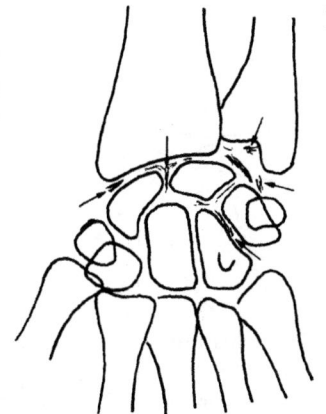

119

120

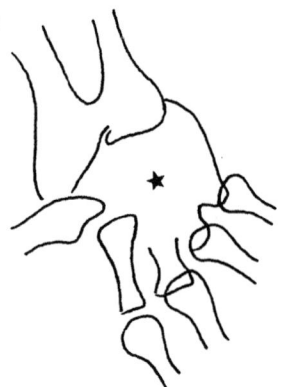

Advanced rheumatoid arthritis.

Obliteration of the joint spaces in the carpus, corresponding to fusion carpitis – total carpal ankylosis.

121

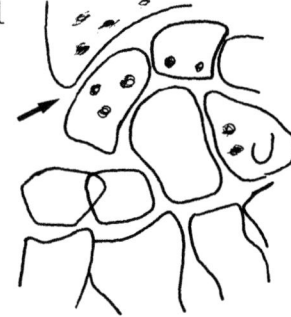

Osteopoikilosis.

Small rounded or oval opacities are distributed over the carpal bones. Their contours are well-defined and sometimes spicular. In this punctate form, the differential diagnosis is from sclerotic metastases.

122

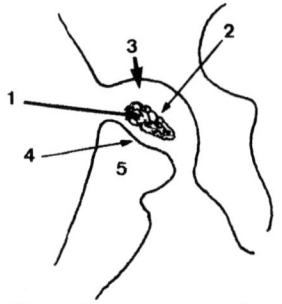

Osteonecrosis of the hip – Legg-Calvé-Perthes disease.

1 Heterogeneous sclerosis of the superior femoral ossification nucleus.
2 The ossification nucleus of the femoral head is flattened – coxa plana.
3 Widening of the joint space.
4 Metaphyseal changes – the metaphyseal aspect of the growth plate is irregular.
5 Broad and short femoral neck.

These features are pathognomonic of Legg-Calvé-Perthes disease, or juvenile osteochondrosis. Early treatment leads to complete healing; untreated, the disease leads to osteoarthritis of the hip.

Talotibial osteoarthritis.

1 Compact, lamellar periosteal bone deposition on the lateral margin of the tibial diaphysis.
2 Erosions with ill-defined margins in the lateral malleolus and the lateral aspect of the talus.
3 Moderate widening of the talotibial space.

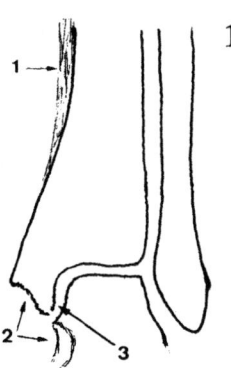

123

Hypertrophic osteoarthropathy.

1 Subperiosteal lamellar osteophytosis affecting the distal end of the tibia and fibula. The involvement is bilateral and symmetrical.
2 The bony structures in the ankle joint are preserved.

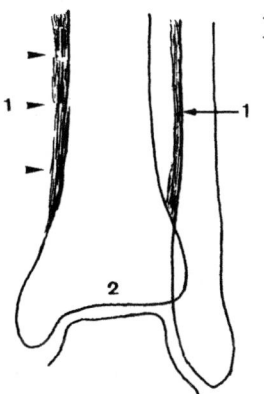

124

Glomus tumor.

Well-defined semicircular lesion in the terminal phalangeal tuft, opened on the soft tissue.

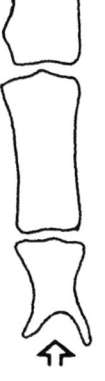

125

126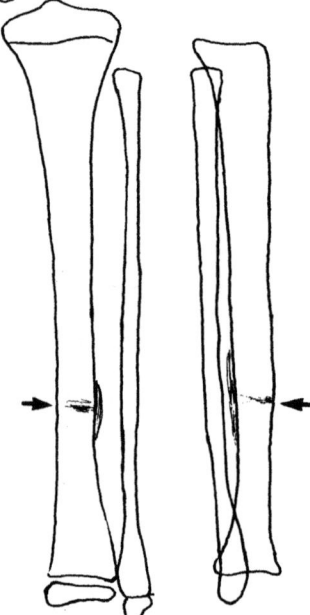

Congenital myxedema.

1 The bones in the arm and forearm are slender.
2 Retarded skeletal maturation – persistence of epiphyseal nuclei.
3 Epiphyseal dysgenesis – punctate appearance of the epiphyses.
4 The carpal bones have a "rimmed" appearance.

127

Stress fracture.

Periosteal reaction associated with discrete sclerosis of the spongy bone with ill-defined margins.
The main differential diagnosis is from osteosarcoma.

Osteogenesis imperfecta (Lobstein's disease).

1 Decrease in osseous density.
2 Deformation of the bone segments.
3 Marked global thinning of the cortices.
4 Fracture of the right tibial diaphysis with callus.

Osteogenesis imperfecta, or congenital abnormal fragility of the skeleton, is an inherited disease characterized by abnormal fragility of the bones, with a susceptibility to fractures.

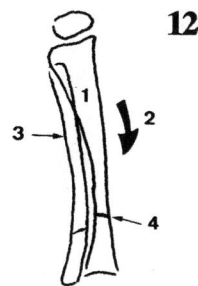

128

Myeloma.

Diffuse osteoporosis with multiple small lytic lesions of the humeral diaphysis. Scalloping of the endosteal margin of the cortex.

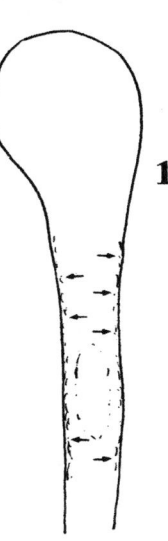

129

Fracture in fibrous dysplasia.

1 Diaphyseal fracture through a lytic lesion deforming the bone.
2 Homogeneous ovoid radiolucent lesion with a regular margin and "ground glass" appearance.
3 The cortex is thinned.

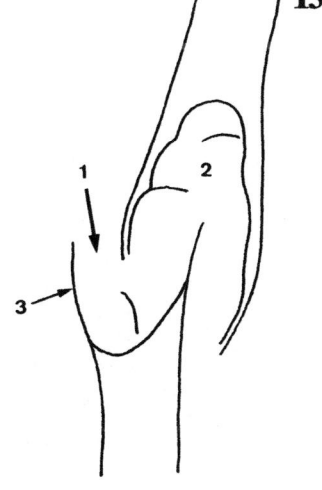

130

131

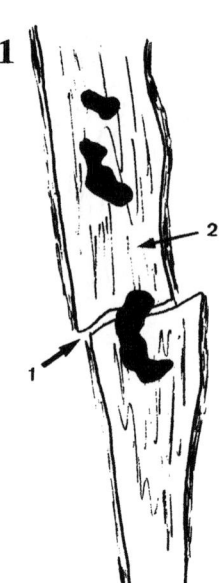

Pathologic fracture in Paget's disease.

1 Diaphyseal fracture with displaced bone fragments.
2 Diaphyseal remodelling – deformation, hypertrophy, coarsened trabeculations, thickening of the cortex. This appearance is pathognomonic of Paget's disease. Fracture of a pagetic bone is a complication, due to the weakness of the involved bone. Common sites for such fractures are the femur, the tibia and, less commonly, the humerus. The inducing trauma is of variable, sometimes minimal importance.

132

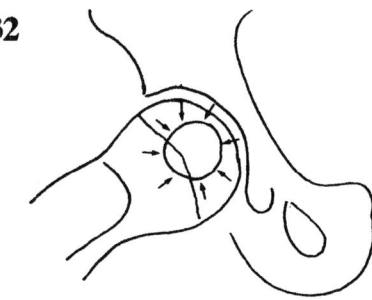

Benign chondroblastoma.

Rounded epiphyseal lytic lesion with clearly defined and regular margins. The femoral epiphysis is not deformed; the cortex is not disrupted.
Benign chondroblastoma is the only benign epiphyseal lesion occurring in children. A predilection exists for the proximal ends of the humerus and femur.

133

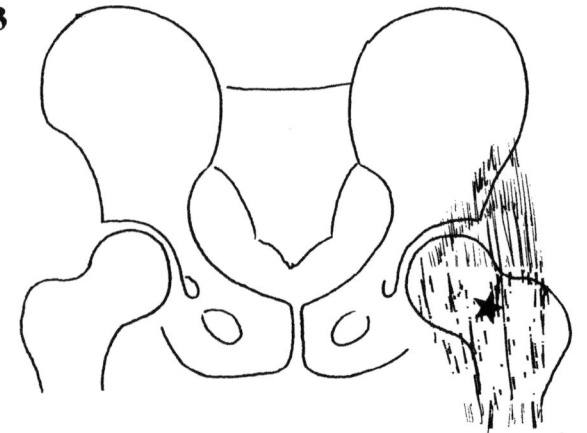

Paraosteoarthropathy in neurologic injuries.

Para-articular ossifications around the greater trochanter. This disorder occurs in prolonged immobilizations, e. g., hemiplegia, coma, and paraplegia.

Osteomalacia.

1 Increased radiolucency of the femoral diaphysis.
2 Deformity of the diaphysis – lateral convexity with coxa vara.
3 Presence of horizontal lucent lines with disruption of the outer cortex of the femur – Looser-Milkmann bands.
This appearance is virtually pathognomonic of osteomalacia. Looser-Milkmann zones occur mainly in the pelvis and limbs; they should be searched for systematically.

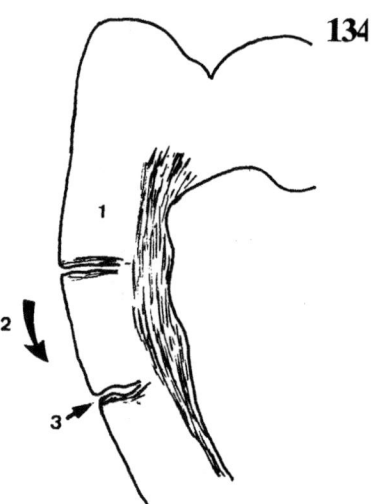

134

Epiphysiolysis.

The superior femoral epiphysis has slipped downwards and medially – coxa vara. The line prolonging the upper edge of the femoral neck no longer intersects the superolateral part of the epiphysis.

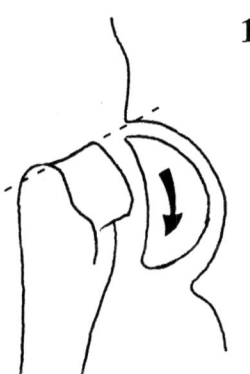

135

Osteochondritis dissecans of the talus.

1 Cortical defect on the superomedial aspect of the talus.
2 Presence of a radiolucent area surrounded by sclerosis.
3 Normal articular space.

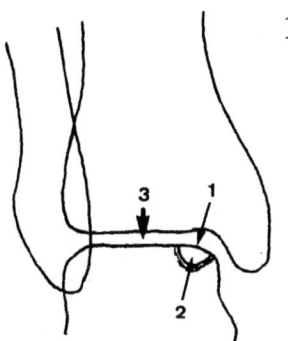

136

137

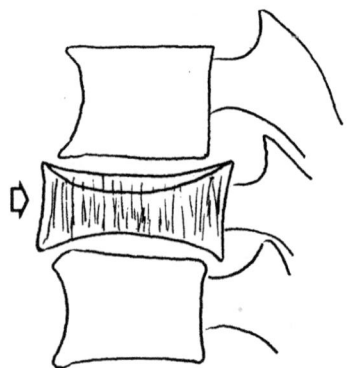

Pagetic vertebra.

The different characteristics of a pagetic bone are seen. Vertebral compression accentuates the increase in the anteroposterior diameter of the vertebral body.

138

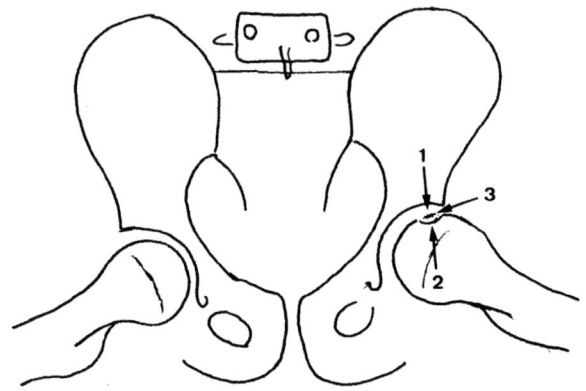

Osteochondritis of the femoral head.

1 Ruptured cortex in the superolateral part of the left femoral head.
2 Subcortical radiolucent lesion separated from the unaffected bone by a dense line.
3 Punctate opacity within the lesion.
The CT scan (**b**) also shows these lesions, and confirms the diagnosis of osteochondritis.

139

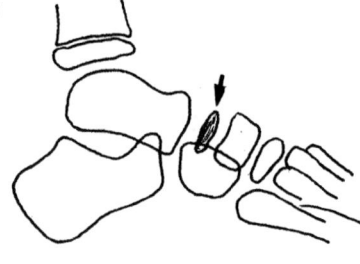

Tarsal navicular osteochondrosis or Köhler's bone disease.

The navicular is flattened, has the shape of a biconcave lens, and shows diffusely increased density.
This appearance is pathognomonic of Köhler's bone disease.

Fibrous dysplasia.

Large lytic lesions deform the femoral end and the acetabulum. Note the association of homogeneous or heterogeneous lytic lesions with peripheral sclerosis.
Fibrous dysplasia may involve a single bone (monostatic) or multiple bones (polyostatic).

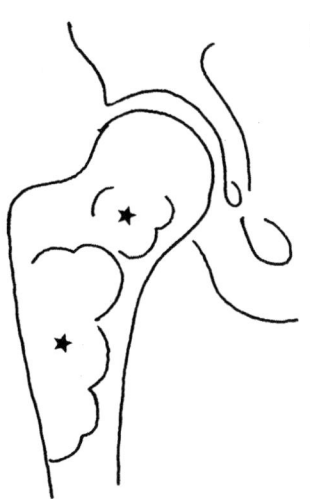

140

Lytic metastasis of a rib.

Costal lysis with expansion of the cortex.
Invasion of the extrathoracic soft tissues, and intrathoracic extension, responsible for the extrapleural syndrome.

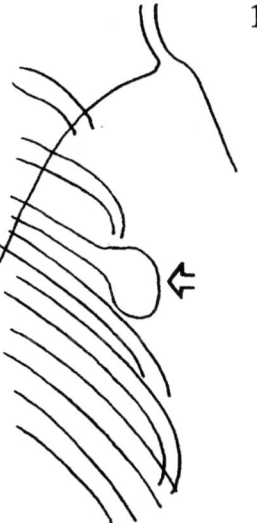

141

142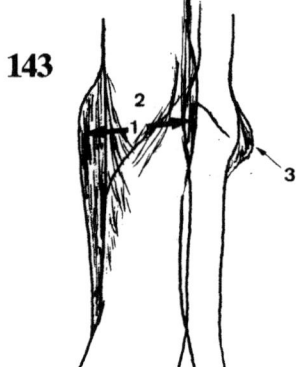

Paget's disease.

Pathognomonic features of Paget's disease – hypertrophy with anterior bowing of the tibia, the bone trabeculation is coarsened, and there is cortical encroachment on the medullary canal.

143

Chronic osteomyelitis.

1 Bony hypertrophy of the tibia due to subperiosteal osteophytosis.
2 Central radiolucent area corresponding to an abscess cavity. A frontal tomogram (**b**) shows the presence of a sequestration within this cavity.
3 Sequel of a mid-diaphyseal fracture of the fibula and presence of a callus.

144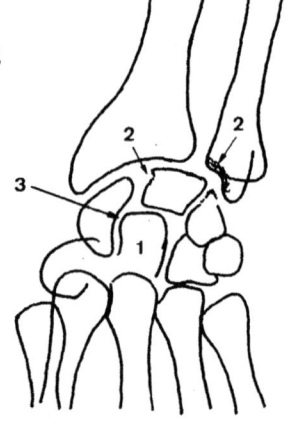

Rheumatoid arthritis.

1 Regional osteoporosis.
2 Carpal erosions.
3 Loss of joint space.

154

Renal osteodystrophy.

Radiolucent lesions with well-defined margins in the carpal bones; thin peripheral sclerosis; deformity of the scaphoid with flattening. These osteolytic areas are due to replacement of bone tissue by amyloid deposits.

145

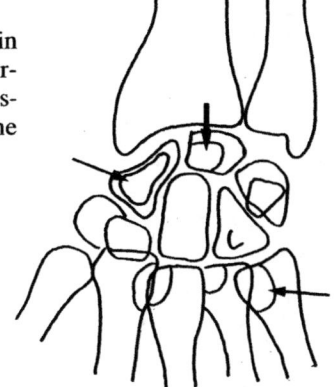

146

Bilateral sacroiliitis.

1 Regional osteoporosis.
2 Indistinct articular edges with subchondral erosions, responsible for the widened appearance of the right articular space.
3 Obliteration of the left sacroiliac interspace.

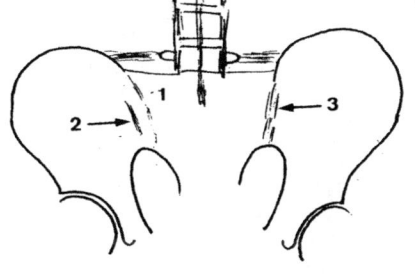

Note the ossification of the iliotransverse ligaments, and the presence of inflammation of the left hip joint. Bilateral distribution suggests a rheumatic etiology – in this case, ankylosing spondylitis.

Hip joint involvement in Paget's disease.

The bone structure in the pelvis is pagetic, with thickening of the arcuate line. Deformity of the pelvis is due to bilateral acetabular protrusion. Bilateral coxa vara reflects the weakness of the pagetic bone.

147

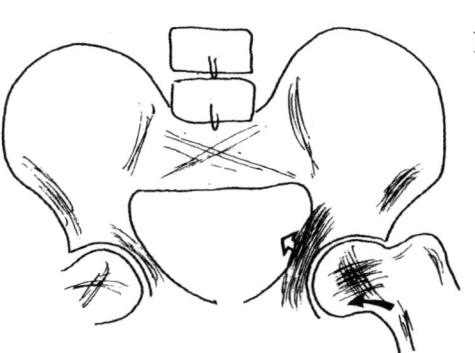

148

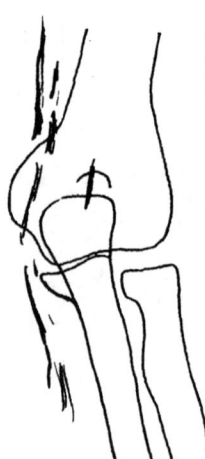

Myositis ossificans.

Digitiform, lanceolate ossification is seen in the muscles of the upper limb in a neuroplegic patient.

149

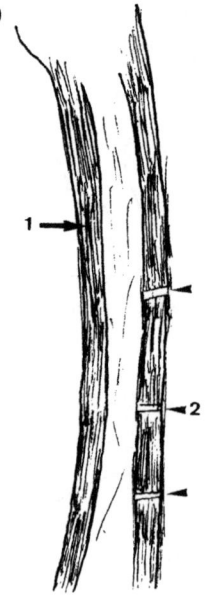

Paget's disease.

1 Hypertrophy, coarsened trabecular pattern, and bone deformity.
2 Radiolucent, linear horizontal areas located on the convex aspect of the bone: these are cortical clefts reflecting the fragility of the pagetic bone.

Rheumatoid arthritis.

1 Atlantoaxial diastasis, reflecting a lesion of the transverse ligament. Dynamic studies in flexion and extension show the extent of movement of the odontoid process.

2 Scalloping of the posterior aspect of the odontoid process.

Note the C2/3 congenital block. The cervico-occipital joint is commonly involved in rheumatoid arthritis.

150

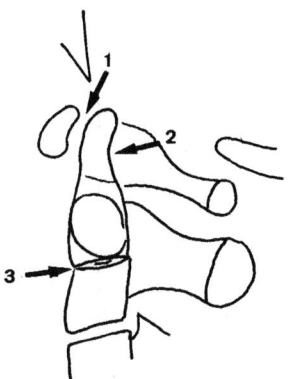

Sarcoidosis.

1 Multiple lytic lesions in the terminal phalanx – "honeycomb" configuration
2 Phalangeal resorption
3 Swelling of the adjacent soft tissues

151

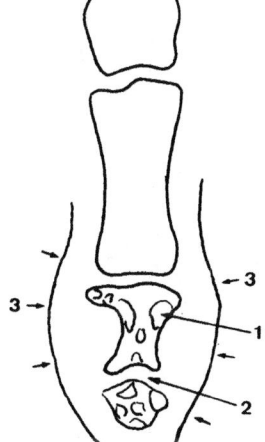

Renal osteodystrophy.

1 More or less voluminous, rounded or ovoid lytic lesions, pseudotumoral, with well-defined and regular margins, opposite the acetabulum.
2 Subchondral erosions in the left sacroiliac joint.

152

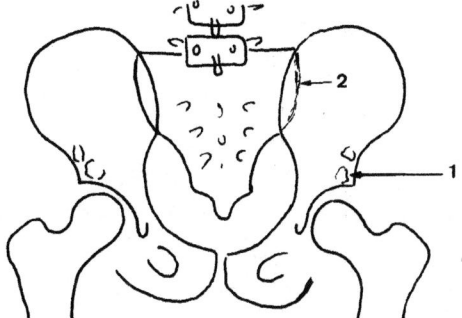

153

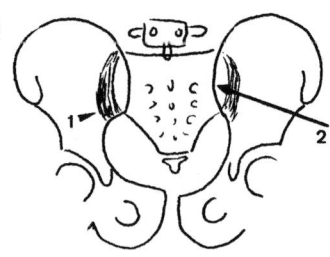

Condensing osteitis of ilium.

1 Triangular areas of increased bone density, with bases inferior, along the iliac margins of the sacroiliac joints.

2 The articular space and the sacral margins are normal.

Condensing osteitis of the ilium is a degenerative disease often discovered in young women complaining about persistent uni- or bilateral pain in the buttocks after parturition. The radiological features may regress or persist indefinitely.

154

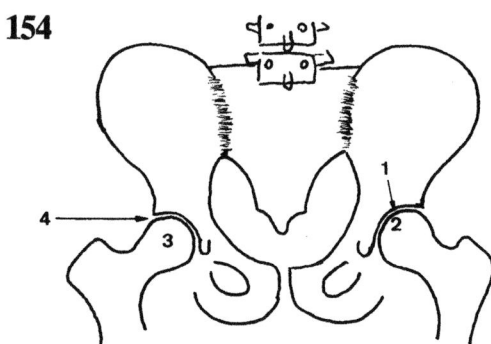

Ankylosing spondylitis.

1 Global narrowing of the joint space in both hips.

2 Subchondral bone demineralization.

3 Femoral heads and acetabuli are preserved.

4 Absence of osteophytes.

These four features are characteristic of bilateral inflammation of the hip joint, occurring here in a case of ankylosing spondylitis.

155

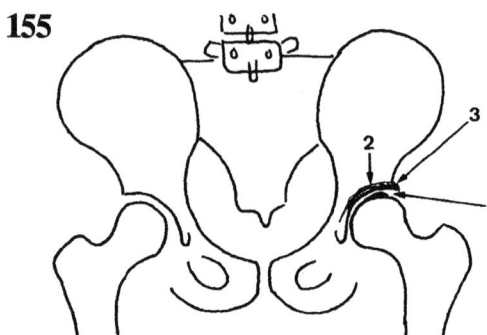

Onset of osteoarthritis of the hip.

1 Superior joint space narrowing in the left hip.

2 Subchondral sclerosis.

3 Onset of osteophytosis.

This configuration in the left hip is characteristic of the onset of osteoarthrosis. Compare with the contralateral normal configuration.

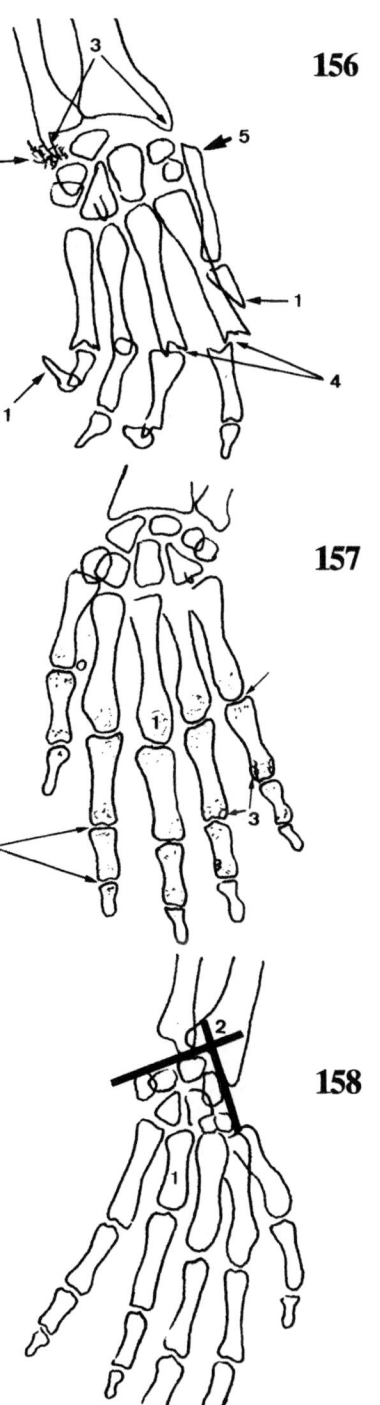

Scleroderma.   **156**

1 Osteolysis of the extremities of the distal
  phalanges, which become pointed.
2 Rounded, homogeneous areas of calcification in the soft tissues.
3 Osteolysis of the ulnar and radial styloid
  processes.
4 Destruction of the metacarpophalangeal
  and interphalangeal articulations, with dis-
  alignment.
5 Bilateral trapezometacarpal subluxation.

Rheumatoid arthritis.   **157**

1 Periarticular osteoporosis in the metacarpophalangeal and interphalangeal joints.
2 Narrowing of the metacarpophalangeal and
  interphalangeal joint spaces.
3 Minor erosion of the ulnar edges of the
  metacarpal heads and in the phalangeal
  epiphyses.
The association of these radiological features
reflects the onset of rheumatoid arthritis.

Turner's syndrome.   **158**

1 Marked shortening of the fourth metacarpal.
2 Decrease in the carpal angle.
These two radiographic abnormalities suggest the
diagnosis of Turner's syndrome.

159

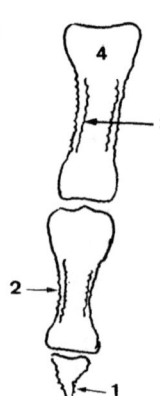

Renal osteodystrophy.

1 Marginal erosion and partial resorption in the phalangeal tufts of the second and third fingers.

2 Subperiosteal resorption, predominantly in the second phalanges.

3 Centromedullary resorption – marginal erosion of the inner aspects of the cortices.

4 Increased radiolucency of the bone.

These findings reflect increased bone resorption and suggest hyperparathyroidism.

160

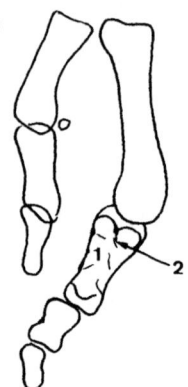

Fibrous dysplasia.

1 Lucent area in the center of the proximal phalanx of the second finger; its contours are serpiginous. Expansion of the spongiosa with cortical thinning.

2 Thin septations are seen in the lucent area.

Spontaneous fractures are frequent in such fragile bone segments.

The differential diagnosis is enchondroma.

161

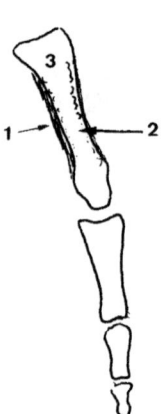

Osteitis of the fifth metacarpal.

1 Subperiosteal osteophytes causing diaphyseal enlargement in the fifth metacarpal.

2 Multiple bone erosions in the diaphysis, with widening of the medullary canal.

3 Regional osteoporosis.

The association of these three features suggests the diagnosis of osteitis.

Interphalangeal osteoarthritis.

Degenerative joint disease involving the proximal and distal interphalangeal articulations.

1 Narrowing of the joint spaces.
2 Subchondral lytic lesions.
3 More marked marginal osteophytes in the
distal interphalangeal joints form Heberden's
nodes.

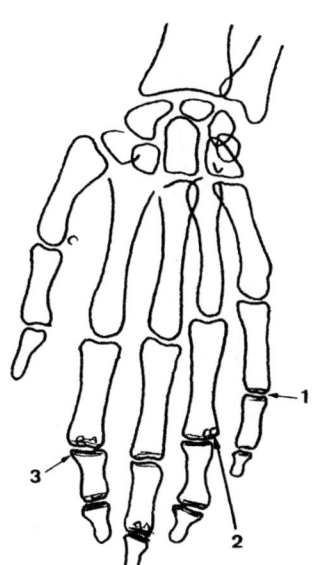

162

Advanced rheumatoid arthritis.

1 Involvement of the carpus – joint space
narrowing, erosions, and lytic lesions in
the carpal bones.
2 Involvement of the proximal and distal
interphalangeal joints – narrowed articular spaces, bone erosions.
3 Involvement of the metacarpophalangeal
joints – joint space loss, destruction, and
ulnar deviation.

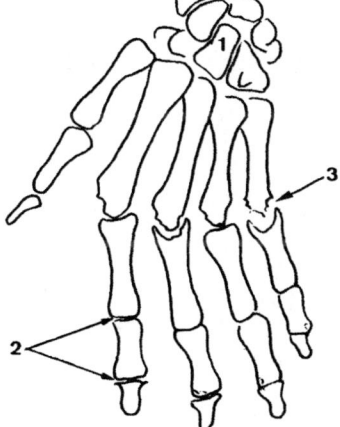

163

164

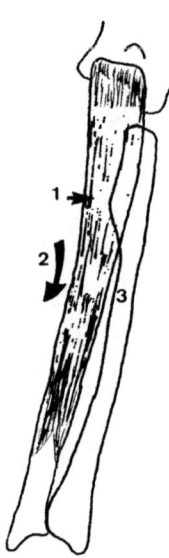

Osteitis in tertiary syphilis.

1 Fusiform enlargement of both ulnar diaphyses, especially on the right, with cortical hyperostosis.
2 Bowing of the right ulnar diaphysis.
3 No changes are seen in the radial diaphyses.
The syphilitic lesions can persist after treatment.

165

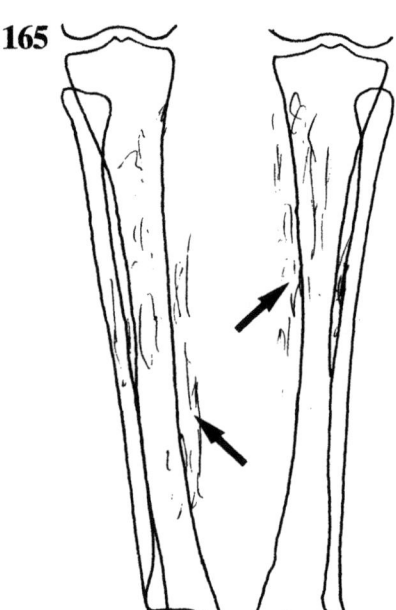

Calcification of soft tissues.

Cloudy areas of calcification superimposed upon otherwise normal tibial diaphyses are a sign of venous insufficiency.

Osteoarthritis of the hip.

1 Narrowing of the superolateral portion of the joint space.
2 Subchondral sclerosis.
3 Small subchondral lytic lesions.
4 Onset of superolateral acetabular osteophytes.
5 Medial acetabular osteophytes.
6 Inferior acetabular osteophytes.
These features are specific to osteoarthritis.

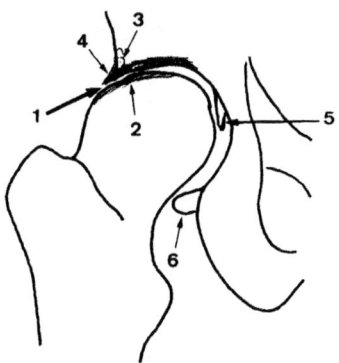

166

Osteoarthritis of the hip.

1 Global loss of joint space.
2 Subchondral sclerosis.
3 Exuberant acetabular osteophytes enclosing the femoral head.
4 Osteophyte formation on the femoral head.

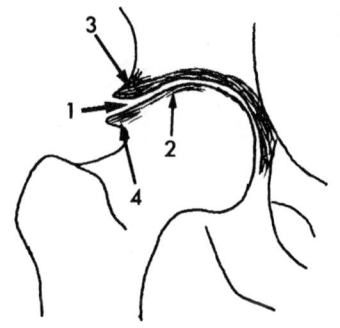

167

Inequality of pedicle diameter (anisocoria).

The left pedicle of L4 appears dense; the other pedicles, vertebral bodies and disk spaces are normal.

The presence of a dense pedicle leads one to discuss: osteoblastic metastasis, osteoid osteoma, osteoblastoma, a Hodgkinian localization, Paget's disease, and an anomaly in the posterior arch (dehiscence of the posterior arch).

As shown in **b** and **c**, the present case concerns pedicular osteosclerosis secondary to unilateral isthmic lysis.

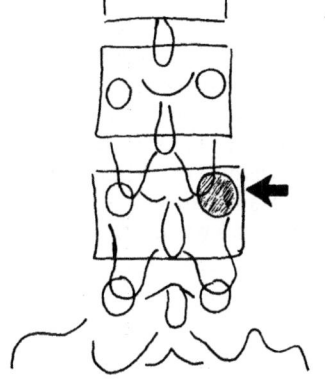

168

169

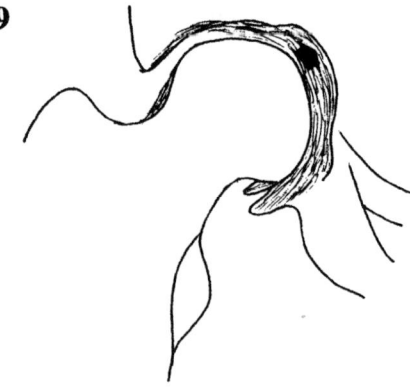

Protrusive and enclosing osteoarthritis of the hip.

1 Medial joint space narrowing.
2 Subchondral sclerosis.
3 Subchondral cysts.
4 Enclosing osteophytosis.
5 Acetabular protrusion.

170

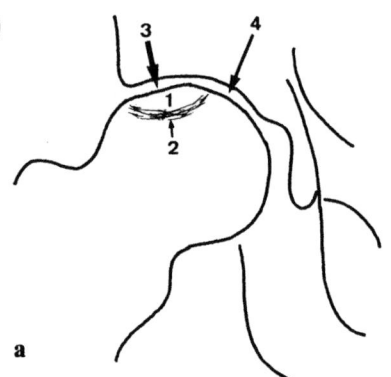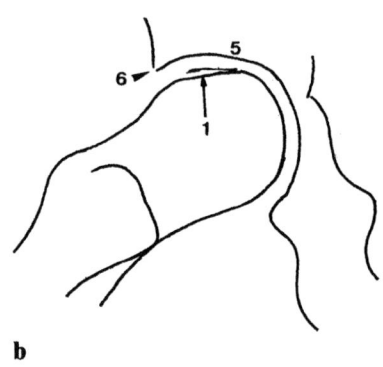

a   b

Osteonecrosis of the femoral head.

1 Heterogeneous demineralization in the anterosuperior subchondral area, with presence of a lucent subchondral line ("egg-shell" image).
2 Peripheral condensation with cranial concavity separating the necrotic from the unaffected bone.
3 Localized superolateral collapse of the femoral head.
4 Normal joint space.
5 Absence of acetabular changes.
6 Absence of marginal osteophytes.
These features are characteristic of aseptic necrosis of the femoral head. This diagnosis was confirmed by CT (**c**).

References

1. Dihlmann W (1982) CT analysis of the upper end of the femur: the asterisk sign and ischaemic bone necrosis of the femoral head. Skel Radiol 8:251–258
2. Edeiken J, Hodes PJ (1973) Roentgen diagnosis of diseases of bone, 2nd ed. Williams and Wilkins, Baltimore
3. Forrester DH, Brown JC, Nesson JW (1978) The radiology of joint disease, 2nd ed. WB Saunders, Philadelphia
4. Genant HK, Cann CE, Chafetz NJ, Helms CA (1981) Advances in computed tomography of the musculoskeletal system. Radiol Clin North Am 19:645–674
5. Greenfield GB (1980) Radiology of bone diseases 3 edn. Lippincott, Philadelphia
6. Griffiths HJ, Hamlin DJ, Kiss S, Lovelock J (1981) Efficacy of CT scanning in a group of 174 patients with orthopedic and musculoskeletal problems. Skel Radiol 7:87–98
7. Maroteaux P (1982) Maladies osseuses de l'enfant, 2 edn. Flammarion, Paris
8. Murphy WA, Gilula LA, Destouet JM, Mousees BS, Tailor CC, Totty WG (1983) Musculoskeletal system. In: Lee JK, Sagel SS, Stanley RJ (eds) Computed body tomography. Raven, New York, 453–515
9. Ozonoff MB (1979) Pediatric orthopedic radiology. Saunders, Philadelphia
10. Posnansky AK (1974) The hand in radiologic diagnosis. Saunders, Philadelphia
11. Resnick D, Niwayama G (1981) Diagnosis of bone and joint disorders. Saunders, Philadelphia
12. Wackenheim A (1983) Exercices de Radiodiagnostic. Radiodiagnostic des vertèbres de l'adulte. Vigot, Paris and Springer, Berlin Heidelberg New York
13. Wilson JS, Korobkin M, Genant HK, Bowill E (1978) Computed tomography of musculoskeletal disorders. Am J Roentgenol 131:55–61

Subject Index

GPSR Compliance

The European Union's (EU) General Product Safety Regulation (GPSR)
is a set of rules that requires consumer products to be safe and our
obligations to ensure this.

If you have any concerns about our products, you can contact us on
ProductSafety@springernature.com

In case Publisher is established outside the EU, the EU authorized
representative is:

Springer Nature Customer Service Center GmbH
Europaplatz 3
69115 Heidelberg, Germany

Batch number: 09635029

Printed by Printforce, the Netherlands